BOLUS BLUES

BRENDAN MCEACHERN

© 2019 Jos. Berning Printing.

Brendan McEachern
Bolus Blues
All rights reserved. No part of this publication may be reproduced, stored in a retrieval system or transmited in any form or by any means, electronic, mechanical, photocopying, recording or otherwise without the prior permision of the publisher or in accordance with the provisions of the Copyright, Designs and Patents Act 1988 or under the terms of any licence permitting limited copying issued by the Copyright Licensing Agency.

Published by: Jos. Berning

Text Design by: Scott Booth

Chapter Design by: Owen McEachern

Cover Design by: Scott Booth & Charlie Sansalone

A CIP record for this book is available from the Library of Congress Cataloging-in-Publication Data

ISBN-10: 0-578-46701-1

ISBN-13: 978-0-578-46701-6
Distributed by:

Jos. Berning Printing
1850 Dalton Avenue
Cincinnati, OH, 45214
Printed and bound in Cincinnati by Jos. Berning Printing

*For Kirstin, Avery
and Owen*

BOLUS BLUES

BRENDAN MCEACHERN

CONTENTS

1—Summertime Blues   7
2—Riding a Bike   19
3—Reading Material   28
4—Selling Clothes and Scooping Cones   41
5—The Scooper Bowl   51
6—Trashy Wedding   62
7—Finding the Idol   71
8—Don't Touch The Merchandise   80
9—Tang's Trouble   92
10—Mr. Cuddles   103
11—The Zombies Arrive   113
12—Everyone's A Winner   124
13—Talk to your Doctor   133
14—The Witches Apocalypse   139
15—A Fresh Start   151

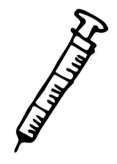

CHAPTER ONE
Summertime Blues

"Zander?"

My body did not move.

"Zander?"

My eyes popped open, but my mouth stayed quiet.

"Zander are you okay?" the murse asked again.

I sat up slowly to see the school murse staring intently at me. He had a worried expression on his face and gently lifted a cup with a little bit of orange juice left in it out of my hand.

"That was a close one, my last day of school friend. Your classmate, Brady, cradled you in his arms and carried you down the hall and into this room just a few minutes ago," Murse Liam said.

I never got around to asking Mr. Liam if he agreed with the title "murse." I heard occasional snickering about him being a male nurse, but he helped me out quite a bit over the past few years, and that whispering was just bologna. Once, he even had to take out my emergency kit and almost injected me with a special but extremely long and scary needle filled with medicine to perk me up. Thankfully, I woke up just in time before he had to plunge the needle into my leg.

"You made it through another low blood sugar moment, Zander."

"Indeed, Mr. Liam. I'm feeling quite fine now." I looked out from his office to see ecstatic kids wearing backpacks heading toward buses and carlines. "I almost made it through the last activity of the school year with Mr. McGovern."

Murse Liam nodded sympathetically.

"We were killing a little time by the basketball court playing Knockout, but my strategy of not really eating a lunch really caught up with me."

"The only thing *caught* was your flopping body when you fell into Brady's arms."

"I hope there are no photos of that. That is pure social media gold." I sat up on Mr. Liam's table and heard the crinkle of tissue paper beneath my sweat-filled shorts.

"I've got to catch my bus, Mr. Liam. Thanks for the juice." I grabbed my backpack and headed toward the front of the school.

"Make sure you check yourself right away!" I heard Mr. Liam yell down the hallway. "And don't forget to keep bolusing with your food and snacks!"

I was shaking my head. Why did he have to use the word *bolus*? I know it means to inject with a needle, but I really didn't want to stick a needle in my arm this morning or any morning just to have a bowl of cereal. I carefully pushed open the iron gate of the Flowing Meadows School and made my way down the street. It only took me one block of walking when the first driver honked a horn.

"Look out!" screamed the driver.

A soda can flew out of the car and crashed in front of me on the sidewalk. It fizzed all over my sneakers. It was a narrow road with very little sidewalk, and people were always yelling or screaming to jump scare me. It made me too nervous to ever ride my bike to school on this road.

I gave a friendly wave back to the passing car and kept walking. My mom would tell me to kill someone with kindness during one of these situations. I was eleven years old but as tall as a ninth grader. Mom kept trying to get me to try out for football or basketball, but I wasn't very coordinated and didn't like organized sports.

I was diagnosed with type 1 diabetes back in third grade. This incurable disease arrived on Christmas morning due to my stupid failing pancreas. The pancreas is an organ in the body that sits behind your stomach. You can't even feel the organ if you poke your stomach hard. Probably around Thanksgiving, my pancreas slowed down. One of my pancreas's primary duties was to produce a protein called insulin to help me when I ate something. Insulin helps the body break down any food to become energy. My pancreas went on permanent lifetime vacation, and this landed me in the hospital on Christmas morning.

I had been feeling sick, thirsty, and going to the bathroom way too much before Mom, a receptionist at a hospital, took me to one of her nurse friends working a shift on Christmas Day. Flash forward two and a half years later, and this bolus of insulin blues happens every day and every time I eat. The body sweat that started in Mr. Liam's room only intensified on that mid-June day when I reached the intersection of West and Hale Street in downtown Beverly Farms. You would recognize me quite clearly if you saw me. I had on a sweat soaked striped t-shirt with baggy shorts, and I drank from a ridiculously large water bottle. My classmates used to make fun of me because I walked with a little bit of a waddle. I'm probably the only one that ever waited for a bus in this fancy section of town.

The bus pulled up and the door swung open.

"How was your last day, Zander?" asked Merle, the bus driver.

Me and Merle, sorry, Merle and I were tight. I had been riding this route every morning and afternoon for two school years. He had heard a few of my stories. I had heard too many of his.

"Pretty well, Merle. Summer started just a few minutes ago. Maybe you will let me pick out a radio station to celebrate?"

"Maybe I will, kid," Merle responded. "Once you check your blood sugar. I don't want you passing out on my bus."

I rolled my eyes. Merle knew about my diabetes. Not too many people did. He knew about my hospital checkups and that the insulin I took helped me stay healthy and alive. He even started stocking low carbohydrate snacks in the front of his bus instead of the lollipops he once offered me.

"Thanks, Merle. I feel fine. I'll check soon."

He closed the door and pulled away from downtown. "Did I ever tell you about the time I helped deliver a baby in this bus?"

I placed my head against the warm glass of the bus and felt the breeze of the air conditioner blow against my face. My eyelids shut for the second time in under an hour.

THUD.

My head shot forward and whacked the metal bar in front of me. It caused a sharp pain to my forehead.

"You okay back there, Zander?"

"I'm fine, Mr. Merle. What happened?"

"Some moron just rode right in front of me on his bike. Looks like he was texting and biking. I almost hit the fool. I would have made a mancake out of him!"

Merle let out his signature laugh, a loud but short "Ha." I smiled for his sake since I've heard so many of his not so witty puns this school year. The bus dropped me off a block from my apartment. The good news was that fifth grade was over. The bad news was that Mom would not be home until late tonight.

We lived on the top floor of a three-story apartment building at the corner of Essex and Washington Street in downtown Salem. This town was known to the world as Witch City. I love this town, but it is too batty around Halloween. You would think that residents would reflect mindfully on the fact that many locals were wrongfully hanged and stoned back in the 1600s. Now, Halloween is filled with a month of too many people bumping into me, asking for directions, and vomiting in the apartment's flowerbeds.

I let myself in and placed my schoolbag on our kitchen table. We had one living room, two bedrooms, one bathroom, and the kitchen.

The apartment was cozy with a good view of downtown with all the tourists running around. My room had a few Patriots posters on the walls and a sleeping bag on my bed. I convinced my Mom years ago that I could take care of my own bedding, and this was my system. If a friend ever invited me to a sleepover, I was ready to go with the instant bag. I didn't have to worry about the light sheets in the summer and heavy flannel ones in the winter. I could just crawl into the sleeping bag on the exposed mattress, and I was all set. It was a bit Bohemian, as my former fifth grade teacher would say about my lack of bedroom decor.

I kept waiting for the classmate overnight invitations to come, but the requests never came. I don't think anyone wanted to deal with having a kid with diabetes sleeping at their house. I was a nighttime disaster waiting to happen, and parents just didn't want to deal with that scenario of me getting a low and passing out in the middle of the night.

I had a few get-togethers this year with some classmates but no overnight stays. I guess I would have liked to, but Squirrel was someone who stayed at my house far too frequently.

His birth name was Sam Jones. He renamed himself Squirrel last year when we watched the science fiction movie, *Flash Gordon*. The actor who played Flash was named Sam Jones. Squirrel didn't want to be confused with that actor with the same name.

"I'm changing my name," Sam said after the credits appeared.

"What?"

"Flash's real name is Sam J. Jones. It said it right on the screen."

"Dude, this movie is pretty old. No one's going to make that connection," I groaned.

"It doesn't matter. When I become famous, and he and I meet at a party, I don't want people confusing us."

Sam reached across my sofa and grabbed a heaping cup of M&M's and popped them into his mouth.

"What was that classroom mascot you had again this year?"

"You mean Beanie McNut?" I said.

"Yeah, that's the one. What is he, a lab rat or something?"

"He's a small red squirrel, quite adorable."

"Well don't call me adorable. My name's Squirrel Jones now, but since we are friends, you can call me Squirrel."

I sat up on the sofa. "Are you serious?"

"Never glance back. Always forward ahead."

Squirrel was always doing and saying eccentric things like that. Maybe his new nickname had something to do with one of his old money-making schemes. He once set up a table in front of his apartment building and charged a quarter to see what was hidden under a covered paint can. He conned tourists all day. Once a patron would give him a quarter, Squirrel would slowly lift the blanket and let them get a peek and a whiff of a beautifully decomposing squirrel covered in maggots. Sam, or now Squirrel, loved it when someone threw up on their shoes. He sometimes had to run away after the trick because his victims became so incensed, but he was never caught.

I went over to the corner of the kitchen to see our old answering machine had the number two flashing on it. I pressed the button.

"Zan, it's Mom. I left a plate of pork chops and broccoli in the fridge for dinner. I'm taking my late class tonight at school and won't be home until eleven. I hope your last day of school went well, sweetie. Please don't stay up for me."

Another night alone. It's a high protein, low carbohydrate dinner since Mom was always worried about keeping my diabetes stable. I guess I'll see what's on TV until I reheat my dinner.

I'm glad Mom filled out that application for Flowing Meadows School a few years ago. The school was searching for a bit of diversity in the student population, but all they got was a bit of economic and medical diversity with me being a boy with diabetes, very little money, and a checked-out pancreas. Being away from the local school limited my time with Squirrel. He still went to my former school down the street.

I pressed the button again for the last message.

"Hi, Z."

Oh, man. It was him. The voice from far away. It was my father.

"Zander. It's Dad. Your mom sent me another one of her strongly pointed emails to remind me that today was your last day of fifth grade. Congratulations! You are now about to enter middle school where the real fun begins."

Dad gave a nervous chuckle that I'd heard more and more in his voice messages over the years.

"I hope you enjoyed that fancy school of yours this year. I guess Salem's public schools weren't good enough for your mom's taste. Although it was good enough for us since she and I both went there."

Dad often rambled in his messages.

"I'm about to head out for some extra work today. I just got the call that they needed a male between the ages of forty to fifty with receding hair, and I fit the role perfectly. Wish me luck and—"

The machine beeped and cut off Dad's sentence. He always had his sentences cut off. Our old tape answering machine had time restraints that he still could not figure out. Dad tried getting me to set up an email account, but Mom said no way. Mom said that all emails had to go through her, and she wasn't getting cut out of the loop.

Trevor and Christine, known to me as Mom and Dad. Mom had stuck around. Dad became unglued about three years ago. He had a pretty decent job at a comic book store, and Mom was a receptionist and did computer work at a hospital. His hours were getting cut just as I was entering third grade. They really argued when Mom pulled me out of the local public school and put me in the Flowing Meadows private school. Mom didn't like how everybody knew everybody's business, and I wasn't spending anytime outdoors. Dad just did not want to pay the tuition.

I remembered trying to read a comic after they put me to bed, but Mom and Dad were yelling constantly at each other. They would wait about thirty minutes or so after I was tucked in with my blue blankie, assuming I was asleep. Sadly, I was not, and I heard too much. The yelling resonated from the kitchen and right through my bedroom wall. Our apartment was much too small to have a private conversation.

They argued about school tuition, money, the apartment. It started off with big things, and then moved to tiny things. "'Happy ten years,'" I heard my Mom say with extreme sarcasm. Dad moved into a motel. Little did I know; the diabetes had already begun. Christmas morning in the hospital. Two days after I checked in, I left with my mother and a shopping bag full of medicine and came home to a permanently missing father. I went right to bed when I got home and woke up to see Mom sitting at the kitchen table with a cup of black coffee and some tissues. Mom gave me a measuring spoon to figure out how many carbohydrates were in my breakfast. I was still brand new to the routine of portioning my meals and figuring out the exact carb count of the meal. I kept waiting anxiously for Dad to come back. He never returned to my kitchen table.

Those were truly unhappy times a few years ago. I heard the loud crunch of my cereal as I reread the ingredients label on the box of Cap'n Crunch on the counter. Dad always mentioned he wanted to make it big in Hollywood. I found out later that his bus took two weeks to get him all the way to Los Angeles. He mostly borrowed money from friends since Mom wouldn't give him any. He called first, excited to be there. He said he had movie ideas, meetings with people, and fame and fortune were just around the corner.

That was over two and a half years ago. Dad had settled into extra work. I wasn't sure what extra work meant until Squirrel had noticed Dad on a television show.

"Your Mom gone for a while?" Squirrel had asked.

"Yeah, she'll be back tonight. She said she would bring us some pizza if we didn't break anything while she was gone. I'm going to have the double cheese with the stuffed crust."

"Sounds good, but you told me pizza wasn't good for your diabetes."

Squirrel reached over and gave me a friendly poke in the stomach.

"It's not, it's a tough food to figure out how much insulin I should bolus."

"Bolus?" Squirrel asked.

"Inject myself with."

"Why don't you say 'inject'? Bolus sounds a bit too medical around me," said Squirrel.

"It's what all my doctors and nurses say when I have my endocrinologist checkups."

"There you go again! Endocosmopology or something like that. It must be your new school. You're getting a bit too advanced in your vocabulary around your old pal Squirrel."

Squirrel turned his attention back to the TV screen and found a zombie show.

"We have to watch this one."

"My Mom doesn't let me watch this one, Squirrel."

"Is your mom even here? It's only inappropriate because it has zombies and blood and guts oozing out of people. Nothing really bad."

Squirrel hit play, and a four-digit parental code came up.

"It has a child block on it. Oh well, pick something else," I said.

"No way! What is her birth month and year?"

I told him the four digits. He plugged them in, and the show popped up.

"Bingo! Such an easy password."

I watched the show for the first time. It wasn't that bad. It only forced me to visit the kitchen once to get a bit of air after seeing some of the zombies rip the flesh off a helpless victim.

"Yo, Zander!"

"What?"

"You have to come back in here right now!"

"I told you I don't really like these shows. It's disturbing."

"Get back in here. I think I just saw your dad."

"What?"

I raced back into the living room and sat on the sofa.

"You have got to see this. I just saw your dad."

"What do you mean?"

Squirrel backed up the show a minute to show a close-up of a zombie. The creature was staring right at us.

"That's your dad. He's been zombified."

He hit play and a shovel came crashing down. Dad's head exploded into pieces of red fleshy chunks all over the screen.

"Awesome," Squirrel said as he backed it up and paused it again. "That's definitely him."

Squirrel played the smashing over and over on a continuous loop. I got off the couch and squinted right in front of the TV. He was right. I had finally figured out what extra work was. Dad was one of those actors in the background that never said anything. Squirrel hit the play button again. I saw zombie Dad get his skull crushed in over and over. Squirrel could not stop laughing and backed it up again.

"I can't stop watching this! How cool is this that your dad is a zombie on this show!"

Squirrel kept watching my Dad get his skull bashed until I left the room.

Two and a half years later, after my diagnosis of diabetes, and having very little money in our family, my dad, Trevor Burke, was still chasing his dream. I haven't seen him as a zombie since that time with Squirrel. I have seen him in other shows as a corpse, a waiter, and a car accident victim. Was my diabetes the reason he never came back or could he not pause chasing his Hollywood dream? I too often think about what he's thinking about, and this sometimes fries my brain's battery.

I heard the keys jiggle in the door, and I popped off the sofa. I had fallen asleep with the TV on, and my dinner plate was on the rug below me. I rubbed some sleep out of my eyes when my mom came in wearing her blue uniform.

"Sorry, honey, late night. I ended up staying to get some homework done."

For the past year, Mom has been taking nursing classes at night to move out of her reception job at the hospital. She gave me a kiss on the cheek and sat down at the kitchen table to notice the three neatly stacked piles of mail that I always made for her. I sorted them as friendly, junk, and bills. She always let me open the friendly and junk mail. She slipped her hands under her wavy brown hair and ferociously scratched her scalp when the bill pile tipped over. I watched her pour a large amount of red wine into a small glass and kick off her sneakers. I came over to her and gave her a big hug.

"Zander, I need you to sit down for a minute before I put you to bed."

I sat down a bit concerned about her serious tone so late at night.

"Zander, honey, it's very late, and I'm going to be blunt. You do know what blunt means right?" she asked.

I nodded.

"We are completely out of money."

"What do you mean, Mom?"

"I mean, I don't have enough money coming in to support us. I have this apartment, health insurance, the car payment, your school tuition, and now my school's tuition. I'm even trying to tuck a little away for your braces."

I blew a little air between the space in my front teeth.

"I can go back to my old school in September if that helps."

"I don't want you going back to your old school. Too many of those boys were mean to you, and people knew all our personal business. You had another great year at Flowing Meadows. A school change is non-negotiable. I pulled you out for a reason, and we are sticking with it, somehow. Based on my single parent income, I have signed you up for a lower-cost camp at the YMCA this summer."

"I can help make money somehow, Mom. I want to help."

"Zander, you are almost twelve years old. You can't work. I need a partner to support us."

"I can be the man of the house."

Mom shook her head.

"I'll start working, and everything will be fixed."

"Drop it, Zander." Mom said firmly as she scratched her scalp. She took in a deep breath and took hold of my hands. "You are just a boy. You are too young for this type of financial burden. That was your father's job, and he is long gone. I'm just not sure what I am going to do."

Mom stood up from the table, pushed her hair with specs of silver in it back behind her ears. Finally, she took my hand and walked me to my room.

"I've already said too much. I'm angry at this situation, but this is an adult topic, and I have no adult to talk to."

"You can talk to me, Mom."

"Yes, of course I can talk to you, but you're not an adult. You are my son who needs to check his blood sugar number, find his blue blankie, and go to bed."

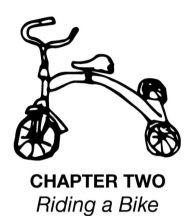

CHAPTER TWO
Riding a Bike

I woke up to see my alarm clock read 8:15. It was the first day of summer vacation, and I wouldn't even have to deal with Squirrel until three. I heard Mom leave at eight for work. I slowly rolled out of bed and pulled my curtains back to let the sun in. The rays hit my eyes hard and gave me spots. I kept blinking only to see floaters popping all over my eyes. I turned around still rubbing my eyes, and he was already there.

"Morning, Billy," I said as I switched into my orange athletic shorts and a large orange shirt for the day.

"Morning, Zander."

"You've been waiting for me to get up?"

"No, I just came in. I was watching cartoons until Mom left. She didn't even say goodbye to me."

"I'm sure she just didn't see you, Billy. She's often in a rush in the morning."

I didn't have the strength yet to tell Billy why Mom never talked to him. Billy showed up one evening years ago when Mom and Dad were yelling in their bedroom. Dad had rented me three movies and tossed them on the sofa before he walked into their bedroom and slammed the door. I'd spotted the first movie, *Spy Kids*, and wasn't sure if I wanted to start my movie marathon with that one.

CREEK.

I had turned to see the rocking chair moving with a lump under a blanket.

"Hello?" I asked.

The lump pulled the blanket down and revealed a shaggy mop of hair with a big smile.

"What movie are we going to watch tonight?"

"Do I know you?" I asked, still holding the movie.

"Are we playing a game? Of course, you know me. I'm your kid brother, Billy. What movie did you pick out while Mommy and Daddy are talking loudly?"

"Um, I guess we will watch *Spy Kids*. Actually, we can watch all of them."

Billy threw his hands in the air in joy. I put in the first movie while Billy settled into the rocking chair.

That was almost three years ago. Billy wanted to know how my last day of school was.

When Dad permanently disappeared, Mom took me to a child therapist. I spent the first day talking to Nancy while coloring with crayons. She wanted to know all about me and my parents. At the third session, I told her about my younger brother, Billy.

"I did not know you had a younger brother, Zander," Nancy asked.

She was flipping back and forth through her notes.

"He just kind of showed up when things were getting bad."

Nancy scanned the room.

"Is he here right now with us?" she politely asked.

"No, I saw him last at home."

"How does he present himself?"

"He resembles me but with longer hair. He doesn't want to get it cut. He doesn't like to change his clothes. In fact, he always wears the same clothes all the time."

"Do you think he's real, Zander?"

"He's real enough for me. He's my kid brother, and I like talking to him."

Nancy left it at that for the session and moved on.

Billy watched me today as I walked into the kitchen, poured a bowl of cereal, and gave myself a bolus of insulin. He winced as I pinched the skin on my tricep and plunged the needle into my epidermis. Billy gazed intensely as the metal tip disappeared and released the much-needed insulin into my bloodstream. I would feel its positive effects in about fifteen minutes. Billy had grown a little bit over the years, but I had grown immensely in the last two years with my height and weight gain. I didn't like to get Billy nervous, so I always tried to keep our conversations upbeat and positive. I didn't like to see him upset. My therapist wanted me to ask Billy where he went when I wasn't around or why Mom never talked to him or finally why he never changed his clothes. I knew the answers, but I didn't want Billy to know those answers. I didn't want him to have doubts about who he was and why he was here with me. I thought if I gave him all the answers he would leave me, and right now I did not want him to go. I couldn't have Dad and Billy both be gone from my miserable life.

"So little bro—Mom said I have to be at the YMCA at nine for some summer fun!" I gave my arm an exuberant sarcastic upswing.

"I guess I will come with you and check out the Y. I have a reading list I need to start soon," Billy said.

"Well, we can walk down to the library after if you want," I responded.

We walked down three flights of stairs. I made sure my apartment door was locked and put the key in my exceedingly thin wallet. I had deep pockets in my shorts that were already full. I had a beat-up phone in one pocket and my insulin kit in the other one. Mom gave me an old phone that gave me only sporadic internet access. Billy stepped first onto the sidewalk, and I felt the rush of early summer's searing heat. I grabbed Billy's small cool hand and pulled him toward me.

"This street's too busy, Billy. We should really walk together." I pulled him in tightly, so we wouldn't be too close to the cars racing past us.

"I don't want you to be a third-grade mancake, Billy."

"Soon to be fourth grader, big brother."

We crossed Washington St. and passed the Bewitched statue of Elizabeth Montgomery.

"We still haven't seen that old TV show."

"*Bewitched*?" asked Billy.

"Yeah, someday. Too many other old TV shows to watch first. We have lots of summer left."

We walked half a block down Essex Street when we came to one of my favorite stores, Smiley's Comics and Cards.

"Let's go in, Zander."

"It's not open yet." I shook my head.

We pressed our noses against the large glass window to see the enormous Hulk, Spider-Man, and E.T. the Extraterrestrial staring right back at us. The huge plastic characters were dressed in Hawaiian shirts, leis, and sunglasses.

"They are dressed for a summer beach party," Billy remarked.

Billy slid his pressed face down against the glass and gawked at all the trading cards.

"Oh, they have new sets out, and the sign says there is a tournament on Friday night."

"Keep moving, little bro. I can't believe you are hooked on all those silly cards especially with all the comics in there. I have boxes of issues that you haven't even read yet, and all you want to do is pore over Dad's old tin case of trading cards? Have you ever been to one of those card gatherings?"

"No, you won't take me," Billy said.

"Scary stuff, dude. Stick with the superheroes and don't turn to a life of crime."

Billy laughed. He always laughed at my silly jokes and imitations. He never told me to be quiet. His smile seemed to grow even more when I went on a rant. I needed to have a supporter like Billy when I went back for sixth grade.

I pulled the door open to the YMCA and turned back to let Billy in. He was gone. He often disappeared when I had things to do or people to talk to. A woman at the front desk asked me to sign in. I wrote down my name, Zander Burke, in my best penmanship. We practiced cursive all year in fifth grade. My teacher, Mr. McGovern, said to not forget him one day when I became rich and famous. I could then sign a check to him as a thank you. I pushed open the security gate and could feel the frame rub up against my left side since the gate was meant for little people. I sort of had to turn sideways to move past the gate toward the children's room.

"Room 115, down the hall Zander," the receptionist said staring at my name on the sign-in sheet. I walked down a dimly lit hall with faded blue paint. The boards were covered with little kid scribbles, drawings, and a theme of butterflies.

"Welcome, you must be Zander. I'm Miss Ellen." She reached out her hand, and I shook it.

"This is the three- and four-year-olds' room at the Y. I have ten kids in here with my helper Kim in the corner."

I noticed Kim, wearing an art smock, doing some finger painting with some kids.

"Zander, can I speak to you out in the hallway?"

I hoped I wasn't in trouble already since the program hadn't even started yet.

"Zander, I see that you go to a private school in Beverly."

"Yes, Flowing Meadows. They like to call it an independent school. It sounds more inclusive."

"Okay, well the problem is that our summer program doesn't start for everyone for another two weeks to match the Salem Public Schools' schedule. You have a two-week head start on the whole city. No other private, I mean independent students signed up until then, so this is the result."

Ellen waved her hand back into the room.

"I don't get it, Miss Ellen." I surveyed the room.

"Zander, you will be staying with the toddlers for the first two weeks until the official summer program begins. We don't have anywhere to send you. The center will have lots of options for you."

I couldn't believe it. Stuck with three- and four-year-olds for two weeks. I could hear the screaming increase even outside in the hallway, and it was only nine a.m. A bead of sweat formed on my brow. My heart raced a little bit quicker. I was so hoping for a stress-free day.

"We'll make the time go by. It will be fun," Ms. Ellen said.

I walked into the toddler room. A small boy with dark curly hair scrutinized me. I must have seemed like a giant to him with my height, orange shorts, and orange shirt, or more like a pumpkin.

Some kids played on a racetrack; another child sat in a corner picking his nose and examining his discovery. I felt a tugging at my shorts.

"Want to play?"

I lowered my head to see a boy wearing a smock. He handed one to me. I pulled it over my head. The smock fit after I jammed my head through it. It came down to just below my chest, but I was able to tie it in back.

"Can you come down here with me?"

I knelt and decided to sit on the carpet.

"I'm Charlie, who are you?"

"I'm Zander. I'm visiting today. What is this thing?"

"It's the water table. You scoop things up or play boats in it until the teacher tells us it's time to clean up and switch activities."

"So, let me get this straight, Charlie. I use this scooper here and watch the water come out the bottom. Or I play with this boat for a while to see if it sinks. I can even pour water down the slide here."

"Exactly," said the wide-eyed Charlie.

"And I keep playing until Miss Ellen tells us to switch to another station?"

"Yes, very good, you are getting it." Charlie gave me a big thumbs up.

I played with Charlie for most of the morning, moving from station to station. He wanted to have a puppet show of *The Very Hungry Caterpillar* by Eric Carle. I wanted to reenact scenes from *The Hobbit*. We settled on the caterpillar. I was able to go out for morning play after I helped wipe down the tables and finish my paper cup of goldfish and pretzels. I had a few races with kids using tiny red tricycles. Well, it was tough for me to wedge my body onto one of the tricycles with my legs bent way out to get my feet latched onto the pedals. I was peddling as fast as I could against Mickey, who Charlie told me was the fastest tricyclist at the Y. Mickey and I were neck and neck going down the straightaway. Mickey took the corner hard around the sandbox and was making the return loop. I tried to take the corner even tighter, and my tricycle tipped on its side. I countered the tip by throwing my weight to the other side like riding on a tilter-whirl, but this caused the bike frame to bend, and I slammed the side of my body onto the pavement.

I lay down on my side in total defeat. Charlie and Miss Ellen came running up to me.

"Are you okay, Zander?" Miss Ellen asked.

I still had my face down on the pavement. "I'm humiliated, Miss Ellen."

"You're not humiliated, Zander. You gave them a great show, and the kids are having a fantastic day thanks to you."

I sat up and brushed some pebbles off my face and arms. The tricycle was unsalvageable. Miss Ellen admired its destruction.

"Don't worry about it, Zander."

After lunch, Charlie set me up in the corner of the room and found me an extra pillow. I felt a little dizzy, so I pricked my finger to check my blood sugar. Charlie saw the blob of blood about to drip off my pinky finger, and his eyes widened.

"Are you okay, Zander? Do you want me to get somebody?" He was quite concerned.

"No, no, Charlie, I am okay. I have to check my blood sugar to make sure I am not too low or high."

"Oh."

I showed Charlie the meter, and it read 153. "This is just okay, Charlie. I'm fine."

"Good, why do you have to do this?"

"I have diabetes, Charlie."

"Sounds serious."

"It is. I'm fine. I've gotten used to it."

I lied. It was easier to lie to Charlie than to tell him all the work that goes into living with my diabetes. Too much for his little brain to process. Charlie told me to lay down. He fluffed a pillow a bit and put it under my head. I felt surprisingly more comfortable than I thought I would now with my fluffed pillow. I was trying to take a nap on a carpet. All the other kids had their sleeping bags with them, but I arrived a little unprepared for this naptime activity.

"Zander."

No answer just slow labored breathing and some slight snoring.

"Zander are you okay?"

My eyes popped open to see Miss Ellen kneeling over me.

"You've been sleeping for a while, Zander," Miss Ellen smiled as I sat up and rubbed some sleep out of eyes.

I couldn't believe that I had even fallen asleep on a carpet with the other preschoolers and saw everyone hovering around me. I followed Charlie out to the playground in the afternoon. Charlie stopped at the exit gate, and I kept walking. I stepped back and waved to Charlie. I slipped around the corner and headed back down Essex Street.

"How did it go?" Billy asked.

"I was stuck with kids younger than you all day."

"That bad?"

"It wasn't too bad, but I just can't do it every day. I'm not going back," I said.

"How are you going to do that? Won't Mom check in on you?"

"Oh, I will check in tomorrow, but I'm not going to stay checked in. I've got something else to do."

"What's that, Zander? What are you going to do?" Billy asked.

"I'm working on it, little dude."

I stopped at the front window of Smiley's Comics and saw the statue of Superman staring at me. His sculpted arms were bent at the elbows with pointed knuckles resting on his hips. The Kryptonian orphan had his chest puffed out heroically ready to take on any evildoer. I mimicked the poise in the window and caught a partial reflection on the glass. I could see a hint of my orange shirt but mostly my grumbling stomach contrasting against Superman's Kryptonian abdomen of steel.

"What are you thinking about right now, Zander?" Billy gave me a slight tug on my shirt.

"Mom is desperate for help. She told me not to get involved, but we are almost out of money, and we need some quick cash. So, hanging around playing with a water table and taking long naps isn't going to help us. I need a job."

"A job? Aren't you too young to work, Zander? You are only eleven."

"I know I'm eleven. You know I'm eleven, but no adult in this town knows I'm eleven. Have you looked at me lately, Billy?"

I focused on the reflection in the mirror again. I didn't see Billy's reflection.

"I can easily pass as sixteen years old. I've got the height and size to pull this stunt off. I just have to act and talk a little bit older with a dollop of swagger."

I stood up straight, tightened my stomach, and pulled the door open. I stepped into a fluorescent comic wonderland.

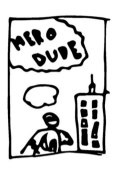

CHAPTER THREE
Reading Material

No Billy. He's always gone when other people are present. Maybe he doesn't want to see me tell a lie and get in trouble. I must do this. Mom can't be a crazy person all summer and support me. Dad has never sent any money and probably never will even if he becomes a famous movie actor.

It's time for me to help out more.

I walked over to the front desk and saw a man with the nametag "Pat" on it.

"Welcome to Smiley's Comics! Can I help you, young sir?" Pat said.

Pat examined me and gave a pleasant smile while holding a tall stack of comics.

"I'd like a job, Mr. Pat. Nothing big, maybe stocking, re-shelving, or bagging and boarding?"

"I'm impressed. You know all the lingo Mr..."

"Burke, Zander Burke."

I stuck out my hand, and Pat shook it firmly.

"How old are you Mr. Burke?"

"Sixteen, and I just started summer vacation."

Mr. Pat eyed me suspiciously while sizing me up and down. I added to my fictional background story.

"I go to a private high school, and we get out a bit earlier than public schools."

"Early jump on summer," said Pat.

"You know what they say, the more you pay the less you stay," I responded.

Pat nodded up and down and accepted my new age. I breathed a sigh of relief hoping this was my ticket out of the YMCA toddler program.

"Yes, early jump. I'm just looking to help a little bit. I've been a lifelong comic book fan and thought this would be a good fit."

"Okay, fill out this form, and I'll show you around."

Pat reached under the counter and produced a job application form. Mr. McGovern was correct when he did not want us to give up on cursive. The form asked for my signature at the bottom of it. I was itching to sign it since I had practiced it all school year, and this was an official document.

I filled out all the information and only fudged my birthdate by subtracting a few years. I committed my first lie of the summer, hesitated slightly, and then signed below the statement that read, "All information is correct to my knowledge."

Mom never really had many heart-to-heart conversations with me, and I could tell she was desperate. This was my chance to finally make a family contribution. I slid the paper back to Pat and let my first lie of the summer emerge from my mouth. Pat showed me the front of the store filled with action figures, robots, and trading cards.

"Let me show you around." Pat waved me down the center aisle of the store.

"People buy those things?" I pointed to the unopened Happy Meal toys.

"People will buy anything if it's priced right, and you make someone believe you can't live without it. You would be stupefied at what people collect. Gaze upon these unopened collector's cereal boxes I am selling."

I couldn't believe people paid for expired cereal you couldn't even eat.

I saw the new comics along the walls and the old ones hanging from the ceiling.

"How long have you been into comics?" Pat asked.

"As long as I could read. My dad gave me his, and I buy them occasionally. My mom wants me reading more and spending less time online."

"Good, video and online games have really hurt the comic book business. We need more high-schoolers like you coming in every week getting the books. I don't want to close my store like my buddies. Some even had to move back to live with their parents. You haven't met my mother but believe me, I don't want to live with my mother again. It's important that I keep up with what's trending, Instagram, Snapchat, and what young people are chatting about."

I nodded and tried to demonstrate empathy. After listening to Pat talk about his mother, I was too nervous to think what would happen if he ever called my mother. Mom would spill the chili beans on me being an incoming middle-schooler and not a current high-schooler. Enormous difference in age. I needed to be highly attentive to Pat, so he would not call my stressed-out but loveable mother.

"So here we are in the back of the store, Zander."

Pat slowly pulled back a thick black curtain.

I peeked in to see rows and rows of long white cardboard boxes filled with comic books. There was a narrow passageway running down the middle of the room with boxes of comics piled on each side almost up to the ceiling. Some of the stacked boxes were leaning a bit too much.

"This down-and-out guy came in a few weeks ago and sold me his entire collection. I took everything for a great discount by paying him cash. I didn't ask any questions. He was dripping from his forehead like he was in real trouble, and I unloaded his entire van. I haven't even opened half of these boxes. I checked the first box in front of the sweaty stranger and knew it was a good enough collection to make a lightning fast decision and buy the whole lot. Zander, that's what you must do in life. Make fast decisions and don't second guess yourself."

Pat snapped his fingers near my face, and it brought me back into focus.

There were too many boxes to count. The room smelled like a wet chinchilla.

"I was hoping to open up this room next week to make it available for all the summer tourists, but there's too much to be done. I'm way behind schedule."

"I can't believe you bought all of this and don't know what's in it."

"This room is what happens when comic collectors, mostly men of my age in their forties or fifties, run out of money, get divorced, or go to prison. When even one or, worse yet, all those things happen in life, I am often the recipient of an entire comic book collection. It's the land of Lost Childhood. You, Mr. Zander, will be the proud ruler of this land starting right now if you wish to accept your title."

"What do you mean?"

"I mean I'm going to pay you five dollars an hour to put each comic on a cardboard backing, put it in a bag, and start alphabetizing and logging them with my handy futuristic scanner here."

Pat handed me a scanner that when I swiped my finger the scanner shot a red beam across Pat's chest.

"Watch where you are aiming! You scan the barcode on the comic, and it will enter my digital database. All the older comics won't have a barcode, so you will have to enter the title and comic number by hand. Don't move on to the next comic until you hear the *PING* from the scanner. After the *PING*, I can then sell the comic in the store, and it goes immediately to my online auction site. Do you accept the job responsibility, young knight?"

I nodded yes. Pat waved an imaginary sword over each of my shoulders.

"You are now king of the realm of Lost Childhood. By the way, I pay the king in cash at the end of the day. We don't need to get any payroll or Uncle Sam involved in this hiring."

"Sure, but why don't you want your Uncle Sam to get involved?" I asked.

"Didn't they teach you anything at that school of yours? Uncle Sam is another way to say the United States government."

I nodded yes. It was bad enough to not have my mother find out. I did not want the United States government after me as well for this illegal summer work.

"Sure, I guess." I didn't fully understand about Uncle Sam, but cash sounded just fine to me, and getting paid quickly was even better.

I picked up a comic, put it in a bag with a cardboard backboard, and put a piece of tape on the back of it. I then scanned the comic into Pat's system. The device emitted the *PING* sound when the comic was entered successfully. I finished a whole box only to see to my right countless more boxes. Bag, tape, scan, repeat. I did this routine over, and over. I felt like I was on a never-ending mousetrap of bag, tape, scan, and repeat.

I checked the time on my phone, and it was already four p.m. Pat handed me thirty dollars out of his cash register for the six hours of work.

"I'm impressed, Zander. You didn't even stop for lunch."

I nodded and stuffed the money deep into my long shorts. "See you tomorrow."

I didn't want to tell Pat that I didn't have any money for lunch since I would have received a lunch if I stayed at the YMCA.

I walked around the corner back toward my apartment. I heard the familiar yelling of kids.

"Hey, Zander!"

I turned around to see little Charlie from the YMCA toddler room waving to me from behind a gate. He was frantically moving his arms in the air towards me. I crossed the street.

"Hey, what's up little buddy?"

I gave Charlie a low high-five.

"When are you coming back here to play?" Charlie asked with wide eyes.

I leaned up against the gate and tried to act all serious and official with the little guy.

"Well, here's the deal, Charlie. I got a job down the street, so I won't be able to come back and play. I have responsibilities now."

"Re-sponbilities."

Charlie tried to sound out the long word.

"Re-spon-si-bi-li-ties," I responded in a phonetic breakdown.

"Responsibilities," he whispered back trying to understand the word he was saying.

"You got it, little dude. Have a great summer."

I slowly ascended the steps to my apartment. Leaning to the side of the broken plaster wall, my footsteps became even slower, and my legs felt heavy. I don't believe this. I was having a blood sugar low just moments from my door. This had just happened while playing basketball on the last day of school. A blood sugar low is when my body goes into shut down mode because I don't have enough energy. I needed to have a snack or a glass of orange juice fast. I careened up the tall steps, and each step blurred and swayed a bit. I reached the doorway and luckily our apartment door was unlocked. I swung it open.

"Feeling the lows. Need juice fast."

That was all I could get out of my mouth before I became too dizzy to speak. My knees dropped down to the kitchen floor, and I flopped onto my side. I felt like I was swimming in the ocean. I may have been exaggerating a teensy bit in front of my mom, but it was a great dramatic entrance. Mom ran over with a glass of orange juice, and I sucked it down in three seconds.

"Can you sit up?"

I slowly sat up and handed her back the glass.

"How was the Y today? Did you do too much running around?" she asked with an expression of concern trying to figure out the how's and the why's of diabetes.

I felt bad lying to her, but I did not want to go back to the YMCA. She needed the money, so my plan was a solid one only to tell her the truth from my point of view.

"I ran around a bit I guess. I didn't check my blood sugar. I also really didn't have a lunch," I muttered.

"With the heat, the walking, and you growing, you should try to check your blood sugar every three hours, honey. Your current routine is a setup for trouble, my dear."

Checking every three hours is not a fun proposition. I glanced at the tips of my bruised fingers to see dark spots. I described diabetes to my friends by asking them how they would feel about getting stabbed every three hours of every single day for as long as you could remember.

I didn't want Mom to get concerned about another dizzy spell, and more importantly, I didn't want her figuring out my secret plan and call the YMCA. I knew she was busy, but she was never too busy to stop worrying about me.

"I will be better tomorrow and check a bit more, so you don't see your handsome stumbling son collapse into the kitchen."

"The handsome yes, the stumbling no. I don't like to see that part ever."

An hour later I woke up on our couch to the sweet smell of roasted chicken.

"Ding, ding! Dinner's ready!" Mom yelled from the next room.

I tossed my blue blanket off and wobbled into the kitchen.

"Evening, sleepy head. I ran out and grabbed dinner."

"I thought we were on a tight budget," I said.

"We are celebrating the start of summer, and I got paid today!"

The Boston Market dinner was displayed elegantly across our table. It was endless chicken, cornbread, mashed potatoes, squash, and stuffing. Billy was sitting at the end of the table. Mom made a plate, and she motioned for me to make a plate too.

"Mom never even gets a plate out for me," Billy whispered.

I just shrugged and didn't want to say anything. Billy was getting upset. His small legs dangled from the chair.

"Mom never talks to me," Billy said.

I just nodded. "Delicious food, Mom."

"Make sure you bolus enough insulin to cover all the food, Zander."

"Oh, I did, and a little extra for dessert."

"I didn't get any dessert, honey. I'm trying to be better about those things."

She pointed to a bulge in her stomach.

"Baby steps," she smiled.

"Baby steps," I responded.

I continued to inhale my food and watched Billy with his clenched hand propped up against his cheek. He slid off the chair without it even moving and went into the living room.

"So, Mom, are you sure about me not working this summer? I think I have a great hook up with a job. Squirrel said—"

Mom dropped her fork with a clang.

"Squirrel. SQUIRREL? You mean Sam? Please, naming himself after a scavenger. A rabid rodent."

"It's not that bad. He said he might have an idea on how to make us some money."

"Listen, Zander. I like Sam, or Squirrel, to a certain degree. I'm glad he's your friend, but he's a tad unusual. I consider him even slightly eccentric, and I don't want you getting involved in any of his money-making schemes. You remember his skeletons in the bucket game? The neighbors in this building were furious with how angry he got the tourists. Most of the people in this town spend their whole day trying to make tourists happy and getting them to spend money. Squirrel takes the opposite approach and aggravates people, and you stand right next to him as an accomplice."

"It's a real solid idea, Mom."

I lied again. Squirrel had no moneymaking plan. He usually doesn't plan beyond the next day. I was picking my Mom's brain about how she felt about my job endeavors. I wanted to share with her about the comic store. The lying to my own mother was beginning to nibble away at my brain.

"Solid? A solid plan from Squirrel? That boy is about as solid as Jell-O. He's the type of boy I wanted you to stay away from at your old school. If you want a great summer, Zander, just relax, enjoy being young, and stay away from any of Squirrel's ludicrous schemes."

Mom stared at me intently.

"I hope you are listening to me," she said. "Did you understand my words?"

"I understand, Mom."

I said this aloud to end this conversation, but my list of lies was steadily growing, and I wasn't even done with the month of June.

I returned the next morning to Smiley's Comics and gently knocked on the front door. Pat opened the door and smiled upon seeing me.

"Glad to see a high-schooler get up so early in the summer and be at work on time."

"Absolutely, Mr. Smiley. Looking forward to another day in the store."

"Great. Keep working on that back room. I've got to do some inventory on what to take to the Con next month," Pat said.

"What do you mean 'Con'?"

Pat clutched his heart and fell backward a bit. He knocked over a small box, and it fell to the floor.

"You don't know about the San Diego Comic Con?"

I gently picked up the box and saw two figures. One man was cutting a zombie in half with his chainsaw. I peered closely at the top half of the zombie, and it was my father.

"Unbelievable," I groaned.

"Yes, Zander, it's unbelievable. A trip to the San Diego Comic Convention in July is a must for any comic book fan. It is my personal pilgrimage."

"A pilgrimage is a sacred journey." I knew that vocabulary word from fifth grade English.

"Absolutely, it is my sacred journey along with thousands of other costumed disciples and worshippers of the holy comic book. I will be there at my booth next month. To rent a booth costs me multiple body parts, so I need to bring a great set of comics to make some money."

I nodded pretending to figure out why so many people dressed like superheroes, traveled thousands of miles, and packed themselves into a convention center for days.

"Well, maybe someday I will get there, Mr. Smiley."

"Call me Pat, Zander. You will, but you have to save your money."

I definitely had to save my money. Mom should not have bought that big dinner last night. I was perfectly fine with cereal. I almost started blabbing to Billy at dinner too, and then Mom would have dragged me back to therapy.

I lost track of time working in the store all morning. There wasn't a clock on the wall, and no sunlight filtered into the back room. I came to the acceptance that my delinquent movie star dad really was that zombie getting his head cracked in on that TV show. Squirrel was right about that one. If that's true, Dad really was that action figure in the box. Unreal. Dad couldn't keep his brain together here, and now he was becoming famous for having no brain. I wondered how many times he could get killed as a member of the undead. If it was up to my Mom, not enough for what he did to us.

I left my bag out near the cash register and needed to check my blood sugar. I pricked my finger and put a drop of blood into my handheld device. It read 150. That was a pretty good number for me, but it should be closer to a 100.

I was ravenous but remembered what Mom said about watching my high sugar intake. I reached into my bag and pulled out a huge Ziploc of carrots and celery. The upside of being a diabetic is that I can eat handfuls of vegetables because they don't have too many carbohydrates. And low carbs equals no shots of insulin for lunch. I can take a brief break from the stabbing. I just wished I liked vegetables more.

"Baby steps," I sighed as I dug into the veggie bag.

By the afternoon, customers and tourists were trickling in. Most were adult men and Pat knew almost everyone who came up to the counter. They went right to the front of the store to pick up their "pull-lists." These are the comics that are pre-ordered, and Pat has them put away in a secret spot so no hooligans like me will even touch or heaven forbid bend the comics. I had no idea that Wednesdays were new comic days. All new comics come out on Wednesdays, and I learned not to be in front of the new comics display as a few people brushed past me. Cordiality was nonexistent on a Wednesday.

I saw one guy reading the latest issue of *Batman*. I saw the cost of the comic, $3.99.

"Wow, $3.99. Why don't you just download the digital comic for half that price?"

The man turned and walked away from me. I thought I was being helpful by offering some savings.

I told the next few customers that new comics are often compiled together as graphic novels. I said I read them at my local library for no cost. I congratulated myself. This was an even better suggestion than the first one! I was getting better.

I saw that customer briskly walk away and head immediately to Pat at the front counter. Another guy was checking out all the old issues on the back wall. The prices were over $100 per comic book.

"I've seen some of those on eBay. Check out the online prices, you could save a few bucks."

I smiled and went to the back room to continue bagging and logging all the comics. A few hours later, I was ready to head home for the day.

"Zander come on over here." Pat waved me over.

He handed me $30 in cash for a day's work. I slipped it into my empty pocket.

"Zander. I've got some bad news."

Here it comes. My mother found out I was working here and not at the YMCA.

"This is going to have to be your last day working here, my young friend," Pat said.

I tilted my head like he was speaking a different language. I didn't understand what he was saying.

"Quite a few customers came up to me today because of your comments. You were recommending digital comics, eBay, and even trips to the library? Those options are like a death sentence to a small business. I only survive by having people visit, loiter here all day, and hand over their hard-earned cash to one person, me."

"I was only trying to be helpful, Mr. Smiley."

Pat put his hands up in frustration. "You just can't be saying these things to my customers. Comics have gone digital, and it's hard enough to get people in the door. Thank you for helping these past two days."

Pat reached his hand out, and I shook it. It was over. Just like that. My promising lucrative summer was over in a one-minute conversation. My big mouth was flapping attempting to be helpful, and I got fired because of it. Pat walked me to the door, handed me my backpack and told me to have a great summer. I walked to the end of the street and started to feel dizzy again.

"Not again."

I knew I was low but not that low. I reached into my snack bag and found it empty. I was dropping fast with no food or drink to help me.

I saw a young couple walking by.

"Ma'am do you have a little food for me?" I reached my hands out. The woman shook her head, and the gentleman glared at me. They kept walking. Great. Being judged when I am having a full-blown diabetic low.

"Sir, do you have a snack or candy on you?" I asked an older gentleman. He stopped and gave me a disapproving look.

"Stop begging and go to work," he uttered.

Now people think I'm begging. Don't judge a book by its cover is what Mr. McGovern used to say. I'm having a low and people wanted to make fun of a kid staggering like the undead. Through my spotted vision, I glimpsed a convenience store across the street. I unsteadily wobbled toward the store clutching my $30. I think I can make it. I know I can make it. Green light means go. Walk across. Don't fall. Reach the store. Buy the juice. Drink the juice quickly, and the fuzz slowly taking over my brain will go away.

I poured the entire drink down my throat as the sunspots on my eyes disappeared bringing me back to my harsh adolescent reality.

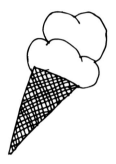

CHAPTER FOUR
Selling Clothes and Scooping Cones

I am once again unemployed. I left the YMCA, and I was fired from the comic book store, or as Pat said, "Released." Mom left cereal out with a note that she would see me late tonight. She took an evening shift at the hospital. I had the whole day and evening to figure out how to make money. I think I am still good at sales. I like to talk to people and be helpful if I can just do it in an appropriate way. I might just have to change my approach.

    I walked by a consignment shop with a help wanted sign on its door. I thought I could be a good sales representative or help the store. I pushed open the doors. A young woman at the counter put down her phone and glanced up at me with her stylishly large black-framed glasses. I knew I needed a job this morning, but I didn't consider coordinating my summer outfit well. I wore long baggy shorts and an orange t-shirt with a large picture of bacon on it. The text underneath the picture read, "Everything's Better with Bacon."

    "I saw your sign in the window."

    "What sign?" she responded.

"Um, the sign in the window said, 'Help Wanted.' I was offering to help."

"Serious?"

"I'm very serious. I need to work and help my mother because—"

"Spare me the life story young tall man. It will show up on my media feed if it's deemed important in my life," she responded.

"I can help out in any way. I'm good with customers. I know fashion, and I'm an expert with folding clothes."

"I wish I could help you out, but our clientele are mostly young fashionistas. We cater to upwardly climbing socialites in their early twenties. I just graduated college, and think I know what I'm doing. The men and women coming in here are in great shape and want to be noticed by others. And judging by you..."

She let the last part of her sentence hang there. I am usually only a bit self-conscious about my clothes or messy hair when I am at a fancy event or a party. I didn't like being judged by a rude stranger.

"I just don't think you will be the right fit in this store."

She waved her hands behind her to show me the paper-thin plastic models showing off summer t-shirts and shorts. I was a bit frustrated over my job situation. I could not return to the YMCA without having to explain to Miss Ellen and my mom where I had been. I couldn't go back to the comic store because I was fired. I needed to vent.

"I can be that cool!" I pointed at her. She pointed to my shirt.

"Bacon is slaughtered food, not fashion. Good luck."

I stormed out frustrated over my latest failure. My friends at Flowing Meadows were probably hanging out at the beach right now or out on a huge yacht. Here I am walking around downtown Salem with my backpack filled with snacks and sweat forming under my armpits.

I glanced across the street to see Squirrel. He must have had an early dismissal from school and was walking home. I walked like my feet hurt, and Squirrel had a bit of swagger in his step as he breezed down the street. He smiled and whistled to himself. I'd be in real trouble if he caught me.

Squirrel was on the other side of the street with a stick in his hand. He was banging it against anything he could find, a trashcan, a parking meter, even a parked car.

I turned my face away from the street hoping he would not see me. Squirrel swung his stick around and annoyed a mother pushing a child in a stroller. I couldn't chance it anymore. Squirrel could blow my whole summer plan. I turned to my left and pushed the door in. The change from direct sunlight to florescent hit my eyes hard.

"Welcome to the Witch's Scoop, young sir."

I had entered an ice cream shop. There were stools and a long table facing the street. I could see Squirrel standing out there waving his stick. He was drumming on some metal trashcans. I had to stay in here awhile. I viewed the menu to see all the ice cream flavors. I felt a bit hungry, and I hadn't had ice cream in a while. Low fat ice cream was often low in carbohydrates, but it wasn't a healthy choice as a lunch option. I went up to the counter and saw the nametag "Dan."

"Hi Dan, I would like a small cup of your low-fat chocolate chip with sprinkles on it."

"Sounds good," he responded with a smile.

I surveyed the storefront to see all the witch mugs, hats, and shirts. It didn't surprise me to see another store making money off almost 400-year-old witch hangings. Dan handed me the bowl of ice cream, and I took a seat away from the window. I pulled out my meter to finger prick. I pricked it once and gave my finger a good squeeze. I was squeezing and squeezing but couldn't get a good glob of blood to test my number. I tossed the meter on the table in frustration. Dan moved to the front of the store and was wiping down another table. I noticed he was looking at me. Often adults reacted in horror or were intrusive when they saw me drawing blood or injecting myself. I told them I had diabetes. One person commented that I got it because I didn't eat well. I politely told him that my eating had nothing to do with my type 1 diabetes. My grandfather had it, and I was told I was eventually going to get it no matter what I did or ate. It was just a question of when the disease would start. I got it because my stupid pancreas decided to call it quits, nothing else.

I did a second blood check by pricking my middle finger successfully. I pinched a piece of skin just where my shorts ended and drove the needle deep into my thigh.

"I couldn't help but notice that you have diabetes," Dan said as he moved closer to my table.

"Yep," I said in between mouthfuls of ice cream.

Dan lifted his shirt a little to show a clear tube across his stomach and ending under a bandage near his belly button.

"I do too little man!"

I saw his small phone-sized pump and the tube that administered insulin directly into his bloodstream. Dan did not have to inject himself with insulin filled needles all day like I had to. Mom wanted me for years to try a pump, but I didn't want the device constantly stuck to me. It would be a constant reminder of the disease and often I just wanted to forget I had diabetes.

Dan, the ice cream man, just had to press a button, and he received his insulin automatically. The medicine left the device out into the clear tube and dropped right into his body. It was all well hidden under his purple ice cream shirt. Dan reached out his hand to give me a fist bump.

"Fist bump to diabetes."

We fist bumped, and Dan gave a large smile.

"It stinks. You don't have to lie to me. I've had it for as long as I remember, but it's still rotten. You have diabetes, but don't let it define you."

I liked that line. I am going to have to remember it. I reached my hand out. "I'm Zander, and I really need a job."

Dan shook it firmly. "See you didn't even say you have diabetes. Do you have your permit?"

I didn't know what he meant by permit, but I was in no position to say no at this point in my unsuccessful job search.

"Yes, of course I have my permit. It's somewhere in my bag."

"Great. I will have to pay you cash for a bit until we can do payroll. I can give you nine dollars an hour. You have a head start on the high school kids getting out next week. I don't have a big shop, so I don't need too many workers in here."

I could not believe he was going to give me nine dollars an hour. I really could save up some money this summer and save Mom. I did not want to mess up this opportunity.

"When can I start?" I asked.

"How about right after you finish that cup of chocolate chip."

I spent the afternoon in the backroom scrubbing large plastic buckets. It was hot, and I got wet even with an apron on. Dan would make the ice cream in small batches, and it would pour into the bucket. He needed all the empty buckets washed and sanitized. This involved me scrubbing each bucket with soap and then soaking each one in bleach. I had to hold each one for ten seconds in the tub of bleach and that burned my eyes. Eventually, I averted my eyes from the steaming chemical hazard.

I did this manual labor for six hours before limping home. I took fifty-four dollars out of my pocket and put it inside a sock in the top drawer of my dresser. The first week of summer was done, and I had over $100 saved up already. I was in good shape to really surprise Mom and solve our family crisis.

I showed up at the store at ten the next morning. I put on an apron ready to start scrubbing again. Dan came out from the back room with a clipboard.

"Zander. I have to go to the Commons to meet about the Scooper Bowl."

"What's the Scooper Bowl?"

"You've lived in this town your whole life, and you don't know about it? It's only the biggest ice cream event of the year. All the local ice cream stores will be there, and my little shop, the Witch's Scoop, is going head to head against the big kids. I'm hoping to finally take home the Golden Cone award."

"The Golden Cone?" I asked.

"It's the ultimate trophy for local ice cream shops. I've been running this place for years on my own, and I think this year I have a chance in the big league. It's been my lifelong goal to win this cone."

Dan's goal was to win the cone. Pat Smiley, the owner of the comic store, worked toward traveling to San Diego for the comic convention. I guess I don't have a major goal in my life. Maybe that was my overall problem. I'm sinking in daydream quicksand over disastrous dad, magnanimous mom, and my dreary diabetes. I had a summer goal but no personal life goal to guide me successfully. I already feel like I'm underachieving so rapidly in life.

"Zander. I've got to leave for a little while to get ready for tomorrow's Scooper Bowl. Can you handle the counter for an hour? It's early, and you won't have too many people in here. Not many come in for a banana split breakfast. Just do cash only, so you don't have to handle any credit cards. You can be a little flexible with the price if someone is a little short on cash because it's my fault. I will still have to check your permit soon just in case and especially for tomorrow," Dan said.

I was going to have to figure out this work permit situation. The city didn't give a work permit until you were fourteen. I'd used my height to my advantage to pass for sixteen although I wasn't even twelve. "Don't worry about it, Mr. Dan. You are a busy guy. I've got this counter covered. I won't over scoop your ice cream, lose any money, and will have the place nice and clean when you return."

Dan fist pumped me as he headed out the front door. I did fairly well for the next hour. A few people came in. I scooped and handed over cups and cones and did not scare any customers away like the comic book store. I had a much harder time putting the ice cream on the cone because it would tip over. One of the cones almost landed on an older woman's shirt as I handed it to her. I suggested to the next patron to put the cone upside down in a cup.

"It's the best of both worlds, and I can put a little more ice cream in the cup," I said. "I will put the cone on top of the cupped ice cream to top it off."

I was getting the hang of this job and feeling pretty chill about myself. My stomach and sweet tooth felt satisfied since I had been sampling flavors all morning. I didn't have any blood glucose issues all day and was licking my lips about all the money I would save this summer. It was time to tell Mom the truth and solve this work permit issue.

The ice cream shop door swung open so hard it hit a shelf of ceramic cups with the Witch's Scoop logo on it. The bang sent me running right up to the front counter. A man with long hair tied into a man bun walked briskly into the shop. I gave a little chuckle seeing his ball of hair resting perfectly on the top of his head.

A small boy stood next to him. The boy had his legs crossed and was hopping up and down. I knew what that meant being a young boy once.

"I really need to use your bathroom. My son really has to go," said the father.

"Oh sorry, we don't have a public bathroom. Just one for employees."

"Well then, can you let me in? He really, really, needs to go," the dad said.

I leaned over the counter to see the boy still hopping up and down. The boy would go in any second. What would happen if I let this guy in? What if he did something to me or the store? I couldn't get fired from another job. Dan trusted me with his place, and I didn't want to mess up. I glanced back to the bathroom and saw boxes of cups and spoons piled up on top of the toilet.

"Sorry, you are going to have to go down the street to the Chinese restaurant. I can't let you back here."

"You can let us back to use the bathroom. Come on, kid, you are choosing not to let us use the bathroom," he said.

The whole vocabulary of "doing" versus "choosing" something really annoyed me when an adult said that as a correction. It was like when my Mom corrected my many "wants" over my "needs." I waved my hand saying no way to the bathroom visit.

The father darted around the lobby and out the door to see if anyone was near the shop. He then stared down at the small drain in the center of the lobby floor. Dan was going to show me how to mop the floor later and move all the water into that drain.

"Go right here, son. It's okay," the father said. He pointed to the drain on the floor about to be used as a urinal.

"No way. Please don't do that," I said.

The boy shook furiously, and the father blocked his son from being seen by anyone on the sidewalk. The boy dropped his pants and starting peeing right into the drain. The smell of urine shot right up my nose.

"Stop right now before I call someone!" I yelled.

The father put his hand on his son's shoulder. "Keep going son, it's all right."

"I'm going to put the hose on you two if you don't stop."

The boy finished urinating and pulled up his pants. He clung to his father.

"Why did you do that? Why didn't you just go down the street?" I pleaded.

The father slowly and scornfully turned back to me. "What time do you get off from work tonight?" he asked me.

I didn't understand what he was saying to me. I just saw his son pee all over the lobby. The floor was soaked and there was some splatter under the counter. The whole store smelled like urine, and I knew Dan would be back soon. I had to clean up this store or he would fire me like Pat and that young hipster who wouldn't let me even fold clothes in her store.

"Excuse me?" It was all I could mutter.

"What time are you done working? We need to settle what just happened here," the father said.

I tried to come up with a time quickly. "Eight o'clock," I stammered.

"Good. Eight o'clock. I will be back."

He stormed out the store, and the cup stand rattled again. I couldn't believe that this man-bun guy wanted to fight me. Over what? His son was the one who peed all over the place. Now he wanted to have some type of a rumble with me? What did I do wrong?

"That is unbelievable!" Squirrel yelled at me. It was 7:30, and Squirrel came running over after I texted him about my daytime drama.

"Okay, you got a job and now you are going to be in a huge fight in thirty minutes? How much have you been holding out from me? We haven't talked in a few days and all this happened?" Squirrel threw his hands in disgust. "We tell each other everything. I don't even know you anymore!"

"I didn't want you telling my mom about me leaving the YMCA and getting a job."

"Hey, I'm no snitch. I know you need the money. No big deal. What is a big deal is getting ready for this fight," Squirrel said.

Squirrel opened his backpack and pulled out a whiffle ball bat, a Nerf gun, firecrackers, and some water-filled balloons.

"I was picturing guys with rolled up shirts, cigarettes, and switchblades," I said.

"Zander, this isn't *Grease* or the *Outsiders*. This guy wants to punch you in the face and knock you around for embarrassing him in front of his son. No switchblades. Well, at least I don't think there will be any heavy weapons. I hope not."

Squirrel started swinging the whiffle ball bat all around the kitchen. "I'm going to do some slicing and dicing tonight."

He checked the clock on the kitchen microwave. "Let's go, Zander. We don't want to be late to find a good hiding spot."

Squirrel opened the apartment door and quickly hopped down the stairs leading out to the street. He turned back surprised to see I wasn't right behind him.

"Come on, let's go!" Squirrel frantically waved me down.

"I don't think I'm going." I leaned my head against the door to my apartment.

"Are you kidding? When are you going to stand up for yourself, Zander? This guy messed with you, and you've got to stick up for yourself for once. People are always walking all over you."

"I know." I gently banged my head further against the apartment door.

"Well, change it for once. Show this guy you're not a chump." Squirrel was exasperated.

I stood there thinking about the man-bun guy yelling at me. My father walking out on us. The fact that I was trying to keep a job and not get into any more trouble. I was not fully convinced that this hipster would just show up only with a matching yellow whiffle ball bat. I knew I was only eleven, but I had seen enough bad things on television to know things could go sideways quickly.

"I don't need to show some punk dad I'm not a chump. It won't change anything."

"So, you're not coming? Are you serious? You're a wimp," Squirrel said.

"I know." I dropped my head and felt my body deflate a bit. Squirrel shook his head and left. I heard the noise from the TV.

"Zander come watch TV with me," squeaked Billy's tiny voice.

"Coming Billy."

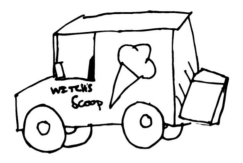

CHAPTER FIVE
The Scooper Bowl

You're a wimp.

Squirrel's sentence was still reverberating in my ears when my best friend said it to me from the bottom of my stairs. I could not attend the rumble. What would happen if I got hurt? I knew Mom worked at the hospital, but what if she saw me being wheeled into her hospital on a stretcher? I'd lost Squirrel's respect, but I just couldn't do that to my mother. Not after all she'd been through. This Scooper Bowl today was extremely important to my boss, Dan, and I did not want to disappoint him by having a fight outside his shop. My money-filled sock felt heavier this morning, as I tucked it into my drawer. Mom always made me do my own laundry, so I know she wouldn't find my old sock secretly filled with dollar bills.

I arrived at the store to see that Dan had already left to help set up our table.

"He's gone big dude." A man in his twenties walked out. He rubbed his eyes and reached out to shake my hand. "I'm Chuck. I help Dan make the ice cream in the summer when I'm home from school."

I responded back with a firm shake.

"You are a tall dude with a good handshake. I like that," Chuck said.

"I'm trying to work out. I've been going to the gym quite a bit. It's helping. Did you see the baseball game last night?"

Chuck nodded affirmatively and handed me a list of ice cream flavors.

"Go into the freezer, pull these flavors, and bring them out to the street. I'll bring the truck around front since there is a prime parking space out there now, and we will load the truck with all the ice cream buckets."

I nodded and headed into the freezer. I pulled the handle to the large metal door and a wave of subzero air blasted me in the face. I walked in, and I was already feeling the cold on the back of my neck. I started pulling items on the list and loaded them onto a pushcart. Chuck came by and grabbed the heavy cart.

"Looks like enough for this silly event. We're good," Chuck grumbled.

I slammed the metal door and returned to the June heat. Chuck flipped the sign on the front of the store from Open to Closed with a handwritten note saying, "Please visit us at the Scooper Ball."

"Um, Chuck. I think the event is the Scooper Bowl."

Chuck examined the handwritten sign. "Oh well. Close enough."

I stepped onto the sidewalk to see a red box truck with a door placed where a trunk should be located. It had pieces of rust on the bottom, and the tires were extremely worn.

"This is the Witch's Scoop official ice cream truck. His name is Stanley. He's been around forever and keeps on moving. Be kind to Stanley, and Stanley will be kind to you. Owner Dan keeps him tucked away out back under a cover. We don't take him out that often. Too old and terrible gas mileage. I think there was some safety concern with the freezer system, but I really don't remember."

Chuck tapped his forehead a few times.

"Someone dropped an enormous freezer on the back of a truck," I said.

"Somebody, sort of did that. Stanley holds a ton of ice cream buckets. It can also hold a few portable freezers inside for catered ice cream parties. Dan and I loaded one freezer into the back of the truck last night. Those ice cream freezers are heavy and even with two people we can't move them well. Close the back door for me, and we'll go."

Chuck took off his hat and wiped the pouring sweat off his brow. He walked over to the passenger side of the truck.

"Where are you going?" I asked.

"Dan said you had your permit," Chuck responded.

"My permit, yes, somewhere." I pulled out my backpack.

"Your driver's permit. I feel terrible this morning, and you can drive on a permit with me in the truck."

Wrong permit. Dan had been asking about my driver's permit. I noticed the dents and dings on the side of the red and gray truck as Chuck climbed into the passenger's seat and pulled his hat down over his eyes. I moved around the back of the truck and bumped into the freezer door as I looked to see cars cruising down Washington Street. I used the step near the front tire and pulled on the doorframe to get me up into the driver's seat. I wiggled myself comfortable and put on my seatbelt. I couldn't believe I was about to drive a truck.

"So, with your learner's permit you are going to have to go really slow. You don't want any tickets on your driver's record. It will stay there forever. Trust me. I know." Chuck pulled his hat down even further over his eyes.

I didn't want any encounters with the law since I had not even started driving officially yet. I used to ride go-carts with Dad years ago before he became an undead disappearing Dad. I remembered the gas pedal was on the right, and the brake was in the middle. Even with go-carts, I was never tall enough to drive by myself. I didn't really hit my growth spurt until after Dad took off. I rolled down the window and cranked my neck to the left to scan for cars. I slid the driving stick into the "D" position, but it was stuck.

Chuck peered up from his hat. "Aren't you going to start the truck first before driving away?"

"Oh yeah, sorry, my mistake."

Sweat formed on my head, neck, and my armpits.

"I know you are a little nervous, Zander. I will help you out. Doesn't your dad take you to empty parking lots to practice? Mine did it all the time."

"No, he's been a little busy."

I turned the key over, and the engine roared to life. I slid the handle to the "Drive" position, and the truck lurched violently forward.

"Keep your foot on the brake."

Chuck sat up now with his full attention and pulled his hat away from his eyes. I put my foot on the brake, and the truck didn't move at all. It was very comforting. I was glad there was not a parked car in front of us, or I would have rammed right into it.

"Push down on your blinker and ease out into traffic. We only need to head down to that traffic light, take two lefts, and the park will be at the end of the street. Easy breezy," Chuck said trying to give me a boost of confidence.

I let go of the brake and put my foot on the gas. The truck inched forward and gave me a snap of my neck as we were now onto the street.

"Easy on the gas, Zander. This is a V-8 truck. Stanley is old but still has a ton of horsepower. Nice and light on the gas. We are not on a speedway."

V-8? What does that even mean? The truck rolled down Washington Street, and I didn't even touch the gas pedal. The truck kept moving. The speedometer barely went up, but we were cruising along. I gazed into my mirror to see a string of cars behind me.

"Ease into the left turning lane at the light," Chuck said.

I put my blinker on and moved slowly to the left part of the street. I saw the green light ahead but didn't want to go too quickly through the intersection. I hit the brake, and the truck came to a complete stop far away from the traffic light. The driver behind me laid on the horn, and I could hear some yelling.

"Delicate brakes on this baby. Just let go of the brake and roll through the intersection."

I let go of the brake, and the sweat was dripping down to my nose. The green light was getting closer, and I was staring at it intensely. Green switched to yellow. I didn't know what to do. I could hit the gas, turn to the left, and make it all the way through the intersection. I was not sure. The yellow light was burning holes in my eyes as bright as the sun. I put my foot hard on the brake and came to a complete stop at the light. The light turned red. The car behind me laid on the horn, and the driver was shaking his fist at me.

BANG!

I heard a sound from the back of the truck. The car behind me was not very close. I could not tell where that loud sound originated.

"Better to be safe than sorry, Zander." Chuck massaged the back of his neck. "I'm going to get a sore neck on this trip, but at least it woke me up. Most drivers always go on yellow and even gun it through the red. You will get the hang of it as you get older."

Chuck didn't know that I started driving early by a few years this morning. The light turned green. I carefully took my foot off the brake and eased down on the gas pedal. The engine roared louder. I moved through the intersection and turned the wheel to the left. The truck moved perfectly onto Derby Street. I saw a wide-open street ahead and took the next left without a problem. I now saw just a hint of green grass at the very end of this street. I stayed in my lane and waved to a few kids on the road. I figured they would get a kick out of seeing someone wave to them from an ice cream truck. I even tapped on the horn.

"Keep your eyes on the road, big shot," Chuck mumbled.

BANG!

I heard the sound again coming from the back of the truck. I pulled up to the expansive lawn of the Salem Commons. It was an enormous circular park in the middle of town. There was a large white circus tent next to the gazebo.

"My girlfriend wants to get married under that gazebo. She said we can have the reception at the hotel right over there." Chuck pointed to a six-story brick building with a golden eagle on top of it.

"Must be serious," I said.

"She says it is." Chuck sat upright and pointed for me to take a right after the hotel to run parallel with the park. I could see the tent in the middle of the park getting closer. Someone with a purple apron ran toward the truck. It was Dan waving his hands. I smiled and waved back. I put my foot on the brake and came to a smooth stop.

"Drive the truck around to the end of the park near the basketball court. It's the only way they are letting trucks drive onto the grass. Try to keep the tires on the walking path to not wreck the grass."

Dan turned around and ran back to the tent. I drove the truck down to the corner of the park near a swing set and basketball court.

"Turn in here." Chuck pointed to an opening in the black iron fence. I slowly turned the truck, and it hit the curb with a huge *BANG*. Chuck and I jerked forward, and the truck stopped right against the curb. I heard a huge bang again from the back of the truck.

"Did I hit something?" I asked.

"No, you just bumped the curb, and the curb bumped back. Haven't you ever hopped a curb before? Probably not. Just back up slowly. Then roll at the curb and give it a little extra gas to get this truck up and over the curb and cruise down the sidewalk to the tent."

Chuck said it so matter-of-factly. I backed up but kept hearing banging from the back of the truck.

"I feel like I keep hitting something." Chuck stuck his head out his window.

"Nothing. No cars, just a few branches, and children on bikes. You're good," he said.

"Do you want to get out and check just to make sure?" I was almost begging. My heart was racing so fast. I didn't want to get caught in this lie when we were almost at the tent. I should have had Chuck drive the truck. What was I thinking? I didn't think I could take any more stress. Stress was not good for my diabetes. I'd walk home. Good exercise for me.

"I don't really want to get out. Just hit the gas, aim for the curb."

Chuck pointed his finger right out at the curb. I pushed my foot down on the pedal and rolled toward the curb. It was getting closer and closer. I did what Chuck said and slightly tapped the gas pedal a little more as the truck bumped the curb. Stanley shot up and over the cement block with a bang. I positioned the truck onto the wide sidewalk. I still had my foot on the gas and scooted past the swing set and basketball court.

"Slow down, speedy, just coast it to the tent." Chuck shook his head.

I heard that loud bang again. Chuck kept pointing to the tent I when Dan waving his hands over to a specific parking area. I could see the Witch's Brew logo along with a few other ice cream store signs. Dan was already giving orders before I could take my seatbelt off.

"We are behind schedule. Get that ice cream out of the truck and into the freezer in the tent and bring the one backup freezer too. I've got the electricity all set." Dan shuffled off after quickly scanning his clipboard. Chuck and I climbed out of the truck. I reached the back of the truck first to see the door hanging wide open. I grabbed two buckets of ice cream and walked them over to our spot. I kept passing ice cream buckets to Chuck until the truck was completely empty.

"Chuck, I thought you told me you and Dan loaded the backup freezer in the truck last night."

"We did," Chuck yelled from under the tent.

I turned around to see a woman right in my face. She certainly invaded my comfort zone.

"Do you know what you just did?"

She was yelling at me so much spit was flying out of her mouth and onto my face.

"No, I don't know." It was all I could say.

Chuck walked around to my side of the truck once he heard the woman yelling. He put his hands up.

"Okay, calm down. What's going on here?" Chuck asked trying to diffuse the situation.

"You know what he did. This guy was smiling the whole time as he drove by us."

I was being busted for being an underage driver. This was it. I was doomed for eternity.

"Are you guys missing anything?" She pointed to the back of the truck with the door swung wide open.

We both gave her no response.

"No answer. Well, I will tell you what you are missing."

She pointed to the corner of the park, and our missing ice cream freezer was sitting on its side next to the basketball court. Chuck and I were breathless.

"My young daughter is over there crying her eyes out. I was just sitting there reading on that bench; Julia was practicing riding her bike on the sidewalk with her training wheels. Your truck appears out of nowhere inside the park with Mr. Smiles driving and waving to everyone. I yell over to her, 'Honey, get off the sidewalk.' She does. This big goof goes ripping by, and then your refrigerator comes shooting out the back door."

"Freezer," Chuck whispered. I gasped.

"That FREEZER almost landed right on my Julia!" She crossed her arms in disgust.

"Ma'am. I am terribly sorry. It was an accident. The lock on the door must have broken off, and the freezer slid out when we entered the park," Chuck said.

Chuck gently defused the situation. He reached into his pocket and pulled out a wad of free ice cream cone coupons.

"Take these. It's the least we can do. We are really, really, sorry."

The woman snatched the coupons and walked away.

"I can't believe that happened. Didn't you lock the door when we pulled away from the store?" Chuck asked.

"I closed it, but there wasn't a lock anywhere," I said. I drove through the whole city with the back door swinging wide open and a dangerous freezer the size of a refrigerator sliding around. I was surprised it didn't fall out earlier. Chuck dug deep into his pocket and pulled out the lock. He was shaking his head.

"With this lock. I cannot believe I left it in my pocket," Chuck said.

"This is not good," I said.

Chuck pointed to the freezer. He motioned to run with him as we swiftly ran over to the freezer resting next to the basketball court. The misplaced miscreant stood on its side with a large chunk of grass stuck to it. Chuck craned his neck over my shoulder to see the tent. Still no sign of Dan.

"Pick it up slowly. It's not too heavy. We'll carefully walk it back to the tent in just a few minutes. No one, especially Dan, will ever know. I just hope it still works. The last freezer I dropped caught on fire."

Chuck and I walked the freezer back to the tent. It felt like I was carrying a heavy sofa for an hour. He kept telling me to use my legs, but it was all back, and my back was screaming at me. I was feeling dizzy and needed to check my blood sugar. We made it to the tent and tucked it right behind the other freezer.

"Fingers crossed," Chuck said. He pushed the plug into the outlet and a towering spark followed a puff of blue smoke. I could see the fan at the bottom of the freezer spin. I put my hand on the metal top of the freezer and felt it buzzing with energy. Dan came by and tucked his clipboard under his arm.

"We ready guys? This is going to be a great day. Zander. Why don't you grab a new shirt, you are sweating. This is the year. I can feel it! The Golden Cone will finally be ours."

I checked my blood sugar after I put on a new shirt. It was a 50, which was dangerously low for me. I didn't need to be flopping down on all the ice cream samples in front of all the patrons pouring into the tent. I scooped out a large chunk of chocolate-chocolate chip and ate it in three spoonfuls. I felt the dizziness go away and my energy level quickly return. It was a free snack, no need for insulin, just a quick boost of energy to get my blood sugar up and get me through the event.

Dan put me near the infamous backup freezer and had me pre-scooping cups of ice cream while he and Chuck worked the crowd and talked to the judges. I brushed off the remaining pieces of grass from the freezer with my sneaker, as I handed a tray of overflowing ice cream filled cups to Dan. I finally had a chance to breathe after I had quite a few cups already filled.

At the back of the line, I saw Squirrel waving at me. He had a big grin on his face. He probably snuck into the tent somehow and was gorging himself on ice cream all afternoon. He already had on a competitor's hat, and a Frisbee and water bottle tucked under his arm. He didn't stop waving until I responded. I waved back and saw a man-bun perched on someone directly behind Squirrel. Squirrel lowered his head to reveal the man-bun father who wanted to severely injure me physically and emotionally. He was inches from Squirrel and holding the hand of the peeing boy. This time it looked like his son was in control of his bladder. I didn't think he would want our ice cream ever again. Did he see me? Was he just in line to find me again? Was he going to tell Dan about the miserable mishap in the store? Was Dan going to find out about my lack of permit? Was that angry mom going to tell Dan about the freezer almost crashing into her bike-riding daughter? When something bad or upsetting is about to happen to me, I often spiral downward in a dramatic series of what if questions too difficult to answer. My therapist told me I exist a bit too much inside my own headspace.

My heart pounded against my chest. I felt like I'd just run a timed mile in my gym class. I turned my whole body away from the line and started scooping again. I didn't want to be noticed. Maybe he would go away soon. There was a sharp tapping on my shoulder. It was over. He'd found me. I was off to jail for what I had already done this summer. Escaping the YMCA camp, making the comic store lose money, starting a rumble caused by lazy urination, driving a truck, and almost hurting a child. I turned around to see Squirrel shoving ice cream in his mouth.

"Witch's Scoop ice cream is awesome, Zander," Squirrel mumbled through an open mouth swirling with vanilla ice cream and enormous chunks of cookie dough dancing on his tongue. I could see some of the chips swimming in his wide-open mouth.

I breathed a sigh of relief. "I just want to go home. It's been another stressful day."

"Why were you acting so weird when I waved at you?" Squirrel asked.

"That guy behind you was the father that wanted to beat me up in the ice cream store," I said.

"The man-bun guy? That makes sense. I wish I knew that. I would have accidentally tripped and dumped all my ice cream on him."

Squirrel took a pause and gazed at his tray filled with a variety of ice cream flavors.

"Or maybe not. This is delicious. I'm going to keep eating ice cream under this tent until I vomit."

I pulled my apron off and put it next to the freezer. The line of people had finally died down. "I don't think I can do this anymore. There has to be a better way, a safer, even legal, way to make money this summer," I said.

Squirrel raised his eyebrow to me, closed his mouth, and swallowed.

"Oh, there is my dear friend. I'm ready to help you 100 percent now that my school is out. You now have my undivided attention. I have just the right idea for you and me to be filthy stinking rich this summer."

I watched as Squirrel returned to shoveling ice cream into his mouth. Squirrel's words about becoming filthy rich were bouncing in my head as I put down my ice cream apron for the last time. His words were good, but the more important issue was they were coming from Squirrel's mouth.

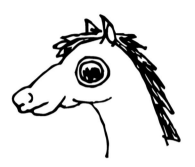

CHAPTER SIX
Trashy Wedding

I have a great idea.

Squirrel's grandiose statement bounced around in my head. I told Dan I needed a few days off. After losing out on the Golden Cone award, Dan just shrugged his shoulders and told me to come back when I felt better. I used the diabetes excuse to get out of work, and I didn't play that card too often. It was the card I could play if wanted to get out of running the timed mile in gym class or wanted to get a snack from the school murse in the middle of a test. I felt pretty good today. I had a new pair of neon green shorts on to add to my brightly colored shorts collection. Squirrel said at the end of the Scooper Bowl that he had a great idea. He went on to remind me of his secret idea many times as he scanned the tent for any remaining ice cream cups. Squirrel told me to get the image of a freezer flying out and almost hitting a girl out of my oversized head.

I stood next to the sign for Dead Horse Beach on a hot Saturday morning. Squirrel asked me why the beach was named after a deceased horse. I thought it was creepy, but many things in Salem were ridiculously creepy. I told Squirrel the story that I vaguely remembered a spooky story about a horse named Wildfire.

"Here's an almost 400-year-old story, Squirrel, so listen up," I said as I pumped my legs on my bike and tried to keep up to his bike. "Wildfire used to be the pride and joy of Salem. He was the fastest horse in the village, and his owner, Jeremiah, would challenge any neighbor to race him. Well, one of those villagers did not take too kindly losing to Wildfire and Jeremiah. That loser then accused Jeremiah of using his horse to transport witches around the town during the hysteria in the 1600s. In the middle of the night, Jeremiah's neighbors dragged him of bed and hanged him from his own apple tree. Just before his neck snapped, Jeremiah watched his barn burn to the ground with his beloved Wildfire still inside the raging inferno.

That barn was within walking distance to the beach we're heading to. The story goes that those attackers and their descendants were forever haunted by the sound of a screaming horse whenever they closed their eyes."

"Time out—demon horse? Hung owner? Horse screams in the middle of the night? These Salem stories get stranger and stranger. Click. Next story, please," said Squirrel.

Squirrel said I was making the hairs on his arms stand up.

"Even today if you walk that beach at night, you might hear the sound of Wildfire coming out of the water and galloping up and down his beach, seeking his next rider," I said.

Salem was famous for hangings in the 17th century. People flipped out, targeted people whom they thought were witches, and hung them. Dan's ice cream shop even has the word "witch" in it. Witchcraft commercialism was pervasive. I was not that surprised to see the beach named Dead Horse.

"Do you really think Wildfire was real and might still be around?" Squirrel asked.

I reached behind Squirrel's neck and gave him a pinch. He jumped. "When you are not watching, he will chomp on your neck like he's eating a crisp McIntosh apple."

Squirrel and I parked our bikes and saw the stream of tourists walking along with beach bags, umbrellas, and carts filled with children's toys. I asked Squirrel if this was going to be a good idea. I couldn't believe I was holding a large black trash bag, and I was afraid I would bump into people I knew.

"Hey, you said you wanted to take a break from the ice cream shop after your crazy driving incident. You had a freezer almost fall on a bunch of people," Squirrel said.

"You are exaggerating. It slid out and nobody got hurt."

"Well, you've got to make money, and this, my friend, is easy money. People are basically throwing money away at this beach."

Squirrel had the idea of going through all the trash barrels on the beach, digging deep inside

large rusted metal barrels and pulling out all the soda cans. This state had a bottle return policy. The state of Massachusetts and many other states charged an extra five cents per bottle when a person bought a certain brand of soda, juice, or beer. You could get that money back if you brought the empty can back to a store for recycling or redemption. It was to stop people from sending cans to landfills. The problem was that too many people threw all their cans in the weekly recycling or worse threw them away in the trash. Squirrel was right that a can in the trash barrel was truly throwing money away.

"So, you go to that fancy Flowing Meadows School, and you know my math isn't that great. So how many cans do we need to get today?" Squirrel asked.

I had done the calculations in my head knowing that each bottle we found would bring us five cents. We had no expenses involved since we both biked down here and were going to bring back, hopefully, our giant Santa Claus trash bags to the grocery store for some cold hard cash.

"Well, we have to find twenty cans to get one dollar. I figure we need no less than 1,000 cans to make us twenty-five dollars each for a day here."

Squirrel started pounding his sneakers into the sand and spraying the sand everywhere.

"Are you kidding me? We must find over 1,000 cans to make a measly twenty-five bucks each? I could make that cutting someone's lawn."

I knew where Squirrel lived, in an enormous downtown apartment complex around the corner from me. There was not any grass even close to him. Most of the neighbors still stayed away from him because of his schemes. "Do you have any lawns to cut today, Squirrel?"

"Well, there isn't exactly any grass to cut around my house, so I guess this is the best option on the table or in the trash can, ha!" Squirrel said.

Squirrel was cracking up and grabbed his stomach from his fit of laughter. He pointed me to one end of the beach, and he started walking to the other end. "We'll meet in the middle when we are done. Take a few extra bags, and we will do this in one trip. Behold all these people drinking their fancy fruit juice, energy drinks, and soda pop. Let's hope many of them just want to toss those cans into our friendly hands." Squirrel was gleaming about his master plan.

I walked down to the far end and saw a sign taped to the lifeguard stand saying, "Tough Kids triathlon coming in two weeks."

I saw the drawing of a kid swimming, biking, and running. A triathlon? This was a serious event, and it was for kids ages ten to fifteen. The winning prize was $100 dollars. That was a great prize, but there was no way I could win it. I was not even sure I could finish the race. Swimming this beach, biking around the neighborhood, and finishing with a road race. I was lucky to make it through one of those events but all three at once? What a dream! I ran the mile in gym class this year or let's just say I started the mile. I never finished it since we had to go back to class, and I would be in big trouble if I was late. I never set a personal record, or a "PR" as runners call it. The ending time of my mile is still to be decided.

I made my way to the first trash barrel and put my head into it. The nauseating smell hit me hard. I turned away from the barrel and dry heaved into the sand. I leaned back into the barrel for a second time but pinched my nose and breathed in through my shirt-covered mouth. This was much better. Squirrel was smart enough to tell me to bring gloves. I could only find the sweaty, long-wristed, rubber yellow ones my mother used when she washed the dishes and didn't want to ruin her nails. My yellow-gloved hands seemed utterly ridiculous out on the beach. I reached in and pulled out a can. Cha-ching. The cash register noise went off in my head as I dropped the can into the trash bag. I found another one and another one. I lifted some McDonald's fast food bags and found ten more cans. Some were crunched up already, but it didn't matter. One was still almost full of soda, so I dumped the black carbonated liquid onto the sand.

I emptied the first barrel and made my way to the second one. I had to shoo away a seagull chewing on a plate of French fries left in the trash. I waved my hands at the white bird, and it flew away. *Beat it.* This bird was muscling in on my profit. I reached in to pull out a can, and another seagull reached in at the same time. The can was resting on a half-eaten piece of fried chicken with ketchup and French fries stuck to it. I touched the can, and the seagull reached in and clamped its beak down on my finger.

"Hey this is my can. Eat the chicken, I don't want it. It's gross."

What was that vocabulary word this year? "It's unsanitary," I said.

My hand really hurt, but I pulled the can out and dropped it in my bag.

"Good luck to you, buddy," I said as I stared at the seagull. The seagull just stared right back at me, unflinching. He or she continued eating all the chicken and French fries. It was gross but getting me a little hungry for breakfast. I saw the next barrel had a can sitting on the sand, and I reached down to pick it up. The soda was half full and ice cold.

"Mommy, Mommy!" yelled a little girl on a blanket.

She pointed to her mother coming out of the water.

"That boy is taking my drink! Why is he taking my drink?"

The girl pointed to me. I was still holding her soda. Her mom's smile turned to a grimace.

"Why are you taking my daughter's drink?"

I could only mumble a response. Nothing was coming out, and I was still holding on to her can. "Can you let go of her drink now please? She wants to finish it."

The mom put her hands on her hips and gave me a huge scowl. Her little angel dug her toes into the sand and flicked it at me.

"You are one of the rudest boys I have ever met," the little girl said.

The sand shot through the air and hit me in the face. I got a few specks in my eyes and a strong taste of sand in my teeth. I bit my teeth down to taste the sand grit in my mouth. I turned away and walked to the next trash barrel. The sand was making its way down my shirt and was going to get really itchy soon. I saw Squirrel standing at the next trash barrel. He was holding two giant trash bags.

"This was unbelievable, buddy!" Squirrel said waving two trash bag-filled with cans in each hand. I held up one bag that was only half full.

"I can't do this anymore. I was attacked by a seagull for taking his or her lunch and some little girl just kicked sand all over me." I brushed sand off my shirt and spit out some sand and rubbed my eyes. Squirrel thought I was kidding, so I shook my hips from side to side and a pile of sand fell to my feet. I told him I could not get any more cans. I was done.

"I understand, tall buddy. Let's turn these in now for our cold hard cash down the street, and I have an even better idea. While you were having fun with that pelican—"

"Seagull."

"Seagull. Whatever. My cousin texted me, and she can get us in as waiters at a wedding tonight at the Hawthorne Hotel. You know that hotel, right?" Squirrel asked.

I knew it well. I drove right by it in the ice cream truck with the back door flapping open and a freezer about to fly out and squash small children.

"Well, she works for a catering company, and there is a wedding there tonight. A bunch of the high-schoolers just called out sick, and they are desperate for help. We will get seventy-five bucks each for filling water, passing out salads and rolls. Easy money."

I was getting the feeling that Squirrel thought all these endeavors were easy dinero. We ended up making only $10.25 each for a few hours at Dead Horse beach. I was covered in sand, sweat, and salt water and headed home to take a scalding hot shower.

When I arrived home, Billy was watching TV, and I didn't really want to talk to him. He was just sitting on the sofa kicking his legs. Squirrel told me to be at the hotel at six, and I didn't want to be late. I put my latest earnings into my secret sock. The crumbled dollar bills were stretching the cotton. I might need to invest in a new banking system soon.

I stood outside the Hawthorne Hotel at six o'clock sharp. I left a note for Mom that I was watching a movie at Squirrel's and would be home late. I would probably beat her home since she was working a late shift at the hospital. I told Billy to turn off the TV and read a book. He just sat in front of that TV all afternoon. I locked my bike to a Dumpster behind the hotel and pulled my blood sugar meter out of my backpack and pricked my finger. The good thing about having diabetes was that I adjusted to the finger pricking. The bad news was I had to keep finding new spots on my fingers to draw the blood. My diabetes nurse educator and my going-to-night-school-soon-to-be-a-nurse Mom noticed that I was developing a few dead spots on my fingers. A dead spot is when your skin feels and can look like hardened leather.

I couldn't push my blood pricker into certain areas of my fingers even if I tried my hardest. A few spots on the tips of my fingers were tougher than Superman's skin. My nurses kept telling me to rotate my fingers and the spots where I gave my insulin shots. I was left-handed, so I always finger pricked my right fingers and thumb. Medical professionals also suggested that I stick a needle filled with insulin into my stomach or even my butt. I told my last nurse it wouldn't go so well if I was seen in public injecting myself in the buttocks.

The meter read 450. I wiped the excess blood on my shorts and now knew why I was feeling a little loopy. I stopped to give a large teddy bear in front of a toy store a big hug when I biked over here. I was having the loopy diabetes highs and had to lower my blood sugar level fast. I pulled a needle out and drew seven small units of insulin from a glass vial and pulled my shirt up just a little. I injected the insulin and knew it would take about fifteen minutes for my brain bonkers to calm down and my blood glucose number to drop. I felt like a kid at the end of a birthday party who has been pumped with cake and pizza. I pulled the needle out of my stomach.

"Hey what are you doing?"

I turned toward the voice and held the needle high above my head. A tall man wearing a hotel tag on his shirt was staring at me. He was holding a walkie-talkie in his hand.

"What exactly are you doing with that needle, young man?"

His second question had a bit of a tone with it.

"It's not what it looks like. I have diabetes. This is my insulin needle."

I showed him the needle and my medicine bag. The insulin vial had my name and the pharmacy information on it.

"It's mine. I need to take some before I go inside."

"Next time don't do this near the hotel. It sends a bad message. We don't want anyone to think people are doing drugs outside this hotel."

The guard turned around to head back to the front doors. Bad message? Drugs? I wasn't doing anything wrong, and I could take this medicine whenever and wherever I need it. I could not believe this was happening. I shouldn't feel ashamed of taking my medicine. I needed to calm down from my rant and probably start a blogging website or a Twitter feed about my thoughts on diabetes and how to survive middle school with it.

"What kind of trouble did you get into now?"

I turned around to see Squirrel holding two tuxedos wrapped in plastic from the Witch City Dry Cleaners. Squirrel glared as the disgusted security guard whisked past me.

"How long did I leave you alone? I can't be your handler all the time, Zander. You know that guy works here at the hotel. And we are working here tonight too. You have to play nice with people." Squirrel shoved the tuxedo into my chest.

"I wasn't doing anything wrong," I said.

"That's what you always say. Let's get changed inside. My cousin wanted us filling butter trays in the reception hall ten minutes ago."

I examined the large tuxedo and compared it to the one Squirrel was holding.

"It's a men's adult size. The suit should fit you fine. If it doesn't just roll up the pants and sleeves and act adult-like."

The tuxedo was very fancy. I was hoping it would go better than being attacked on a beach.

"This will be seventy-five bucks in our pockets and add that to the money from the cans. It will be a great evening," Squirrel said.

"I hope it goes well. I don't need any more drama for one day," I responded firmly to Squirrel. He started motioning me toward the bathroom to change.

"Filling water, butter, and extra rolls. Money in the bank. Or in your case, money in your sock," Squirrel said with a smile.

"How do you know where I keep my money?" I was very concerned.

"Haven't you figured that out yet my tuxedoed friend? Squirrel knows all. Squirrel knows all."

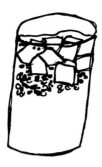

CHAPTER SEVEN
Finding the Idol

The wedding wasn't so miserable. I stacked butter onto small dishes already filled with butter. I brought extra salads to some people anxiously waving me to their table. The tuxedo fit well, and I moved around the ballroom without bumping into anyone or breaking anything. I saw the bridal couple on the dance floor, and this was my chance to snag a dinner roll since I was getting hungry. I felt a tap on my shoulder, and Squirrel was pulling me toward a corner of the room.

We hid behind a beverage cart filled with all types of drinks. My eyes lit up when I saw a nozzle with all the buttons on it.

"I've got something to go over with you, Zander," Squirrel whispered to me.

I was too fixated on the beverage nozzle to listen to any of Squirrel's words. I just nodded every few seconds. The nozzle had buttons for soda, diet, root beer, and carbonated water. I didn't have time to check my blood glucose number and dose myself on the spot, so I had to go with the only choice that had no carbohydrates: plain, no taste carbonated bubbly water. I glanced behind the stand, and the cups were on the top of the counter. Squirrel and I were well hidden, but I didn't want to risk being seen by the wildly gesticulating dancing wedding guests by reaching my hand and grabbing a glass. Also, with my luck, the glass would slip, crash to the ground, and all 200 guests would turn and gawk at Squirrel and me. I did not need that type of attention.

As I pulled the nozzle toward me a long hose traveled with it like a garden hose. I made sure the end of the nozzle did not hit my mouth since I didn't want to be gross and pass my germs onto anyone else. I opened my mouth and hit the seltzer button. The water came out at a decent pace, and I swallowed and swallowed some more. My mom used to tell me to fill up on carbonated water when I was hungry since the carbonation would keep my hunger down or subside it, and it had no carbohydrates. It was a win-win in the diabetes game of life.

The sparkling bubbles slid down my throat as Squirrel continued to babble next to me. It filled me up slowly. Squirrel tapped at my shoulder. I let go of the nozzle and carefully placed it back in its holder. I wiped my wet mouth with the back of my hand and turned my full attention to Squirrel.

"Are you done?" Squirrel annoyingly asked.

I nodded an affirmative.

"Every time I think I have you figured out, you throw me a curveball. You get weirder and weirder, Zander."

"That's your opinion. I was thirsty." I let out a huge burp.

"Listen, my cousin already paid us, so here's your cash."

I slipped the folded bills into my pocket.

"Since we already got paid, we can sneak out early. It's just awful dancing left. The dessert is already out, and people are cleaning up. I really don't want to pick up anymore trash today," Squirrel said.

Squirrel was finally making sense. I was tired, and now I had a thick wad of folded cash in my pocket. He pointed toward the back door of the function room. We stayed tight against the wall and exited the room without any hassle.

Squirrel and I walked through the lobby, and I undid my bowtie.

"I've got to get these suits back to my cousin pronto, so let's go get changed in the bathroom over there," Squirrel whispered as we moved through the lobby.

Squirrel pointed to the door next to all the tourist brochures. I pulled off my bowtie when I saw a man posting a sign near all the tourist brochures in the lobby. We moved closer to the bathroom door when I saw his sign had the word "Zombie" on it. I stopped, and Squirrel kept waving me on. The flyer had a picture of a horde of zombies wearing old-fashioned clothes walking toward a crowd of shrieking people.

"You like the sign?" the person taping a second advertisement asked me.

I analyzed the sign and said, *"The Witches Apocalypse.* It's a cool title."

"Good. I came up with it. I'm one of the producers, Ernie Reynolds."

Ernie shook my hand and made sure the signs were prominently displayed in front of a whale watch cruise and another flyer claiming to catch your own lobsters. Ernie handed me an extra poster from within his backpack. Ernie's name was prominently displayed at the bottom of the poster.

"We are filming here next month in Salem and will need quite a few extra actors for the big chase scene through downtown. It's going to be the ultimate zombie rampage. The movie production will take over the whole city for a week. Tell all your friends to audition as extras."

I saw that the zombies were all wearing Puritan clothing or clothing from the 17th century.

"So, Mr. Reynolds, the zombies are the recently resurrected victims of the Salem witch hunt in the 17th century? This is amazing! Any movie with zombies in it is a movie worth watching"

Ernie Reynolds let out an enormous grin.

"Are they returning to seek vengeance due to their unfortunate and untimely deaths and seeking revenge on the ancestors of those who killed them so many centuries ago?"

Mr. Reynolds nodded and patted me on the shoulder.

"Well, you must be a pretty brilliant kid at your school. You basically just detailed the plot of next summer's mega blockbuster."

I didn't have the heart to tell him that the movie's plot was a little bit clichéd, but it still was amazing that this big-time movie was going to be filmed in my town.

"Well, Mr. Reynolds, it smells like a guaranteed hit. I will tell all my friends in person and online."

"Don't forget to audition as a movie extra," Mr. Reynolds said.

The producer walked away, probably to hang up more signs all over the city or smack his head against a wall. I had enough zombie action for a while. Squirrel came out dressed in his wrinkled summer clothes with his tuxedo in a black garment bag.

"Were you still talking to that guy? Let's go! We have to get these penguin suits back to my cousin pronto."

I quickly changed and headed toward the door that led us outside the hotel when Squirrel tugged on my shirt.

"We have to go check this out," Squirrel said.

Squirrel pointed to a sign that read, "Salem Idol." It was Salem's local talent show. Singers were trying out for the honor of being the top voices in the area.

Squirrel carefully pulled open the door, and we slid into the back of the function room. It was totally dark except for a spotlight from above beaming down onto the next contestant. The room was silent as a young vocalist belted out her next song. Squirrel and I leaned against a wall behind the control panel as I watched people in black shirts press buttons and turn dials methodically.

HICCUP.

The sound exploded out of my mouth. It started deep within my lungs and shot out of my lips before my hand could reach my mouth.

HICCUP.

Another one!

The man in black turned around from the control panel and shot me a death scowl. I was holding both hands to my mouth and suppressed the next one, but it really hurt.

"Cut it out, you are going to get us into so much trouble," Squirrel whispered into my ear. I knew I drank quite a bit of seltzer water but didn't think it would hit my stomach this badly. I felt a sharp rumbling in my stomach and was pushing my stomach in. Squirrel turned to me and mouthed, "Cut it out." We clapped as the next performer came onto the stage. I moved my hands away from my stomach to start clapping for the next guest.

HICCUP.

HICCUP.

My mouth was exposed, and I could not stop the noise from coming out. Squirrel threw his hands up in frustration. The control panel worker swiveled around in his chair and motioned to a large man by the door wearing a security shirt. The control worker made a slashing motion with his index finger across his neck. The security guard politely grabbed me and Squirrel by our flimsy tee-shirts and pushed us through the doors. We stumbled into the hallway still being guided by the guard. I groaned when I saw a second guard in the lobby. It was the same one who scolded me for using a syringe near a Dumpster a few hours earlier.

"Hey!" he said.

"Do you know these guys, Leonard?"

Leonard, the guard from earlier, walked right up and stared at us.

"I know these guys. This one had some needles on him earlier and was monkeying around behind the hotel."

Security guard Leonard annoyed me. "I told you I'm diabetic. I need the needles for my insulin."

"Yeah, that's what you told me," Leonard said crossing his arms and giving me a huge stare down.

"That's what I said. I have diabetes, and I need to bolus to stay healthy. Do you wish to see a doctor's note?"

"Don't get fresh with me, kid. I didn't really believe you this afternoon, and I've been thinking about our encounter all day. Maybe it's time we talked to the police about you two," Leonard said.

The police? I could not believe it. I had diabetes and needed to bolus. We were escorted through the lobby until I stubbed my toe on a rug and bumped Squirrel. He slid to his right and smacked right into a large green vase on a pedestal. I felt like I was in slow motion as the vase wobbled left and right and fell off the stand. I stuck my foot out as the vase descended. The top of the vase hit right off my big toe and then rolled onto the floor. I was hoping my foot would take the force of the impact. I saw the uninjured vase on its side as Leonard was pointing toward a police car out front.

"Just adding fuel to the fire, my friend."

***

I woke up to a dim light in the hallway. I used my hands to rub the sleep out of my eyes and sat up from a bed. Now I could see bars in front of me and an exposed metal toilet in the corner of the room. I heard the quick steps of someone coming down the hall and stopped.

"Zander are you okay?"

It was Mom.

"Could you let him out now, please?" My mom admonished the police officer next to her.

"It says here all the paperwork has been filled out, and he can go home now," said the officer.

"Was this really necessary? He's not even a twelve-year-old kid, and you locked him up in a jail cell until I got here from my night class? Did you review his intake form to see he has diabetes? What if he had a medical emergency in this holding cell? Was there anyone watching him? Do you have medicine onsite to assist if he has a reaction?" My mom was on a roll and furious.

"Listen, Mrs.—"

"Ms. Christine Burke," my mother corrected the officer.

"We put the juvenile delinquents in a single person cell for a couple of hours. It's a scare-them-straight tactic to make sure they never come back here again."

"Trust me officer, I will not be back," I said as I pressed my cheeks against the iron bars of my cell.

"Don't say anything else, Zander. It will be held against you some way."

My Mom was completely enraged and grabbed me by the arm and escorted me out down the long hallway and into our car.

I felt like she was driving a little faster than her normal speed.

"What were you thinking, Zander?" She threw her hands up in frustration as soon as she started her car. It was almost midnight, and Mom was still in her hospital clothes.

"I got a call a few hours ago. The police told me what you did and if I left immediately, I would have lost a night's pay," she said. "I also had to leave my anatomy class early."

"It's okay. I fell asleep after I sat down on the surprisingly comfortable bed."

"Oh, you took a nice nap, I see." My mother was building up steam.

"I did this for you. For us," I responded.

"For me? Being in a jail was done for me? Am I supposed to be proud of you? I am tired of people saying they are doing things for me. Your father said that years ago that he was leaving 'for the family.'"

"Mom, we need the money, and Squirrel got me a job helping at a wedding. I drank too much seltzer and interrupted the show. I'm sorry."

"Too many sorry's coming out of you, Zander. I spoke to Ms. Ellen, the director of the YMCA, this afternoon. She said you haven't been at the camp in over a week. A WEEK! What have you been doing all that time I thought you were at the camp?"

Mom took her right hand off the steering wheel and was waving all around and gesticulating at me.

"That camp was for little children, Mom. Have you seen me lately?"

I put my size eleven sneaker on the dashboard. "I tried a few odd jobs around town, all to try to save us some money. I am worried about you."

"About me? Zander worry about Zander, and I will worry about you AND me. While you were taking your catnap at the police station, I informed your dear friend Squirrel that you are both now listed on the police's juvenile rehabilitation program. Your tough-as-nails smart-aleck friend threw up on his own expensive sneakers when I gave him the upsetting news," Mom said.

Juvenile rehabilitation? That's adult code for hard labor for kids. I'd be making license plates by hand or picking up trash on the side of the road. I'd have to wear a bright orange jumpsuit. I'd be a Halloween pumpkin in the scorched summer heat.

Mom took a deep breath before pulling into the parking lot behind our apartment.

"In your own unusual and misguided way, I do appreciate you trying to help our dire situation. The only true juvenile in need of rehabilitation in our family is your father. He took off, and you were only trying to help. The city put you on their juvenile delinquent watch list to straighten you out fast. They don't want any more trouble out of you or Squirrel. I spoke to the officer, and he knows you are a good kid. A potentially great kid. You attend an excellent school, earn high marks, and you've made a few ridiculous mistakes recently. The program will now force you to help the city. It will allow you to think about others for a while."

Mom and I exited our car. It was a full moon out and great to be back home. The image of being fitted for an orange jump suit crystallized in my head.

"I signed you up for the ranger guide program. The police had quite a selection of programs ranging from sweeping the roads to scrubbing bathrooms at the beach. I chose the city ranger program because of your love of history," Mom said.

I scrunched my brow. "I'm not sure what a park ranger is, Mom."

"I guess we haven't been on a day trip in a while. You are assigned to start at the House of Seven Gables the day after tomorrow. You have some cramming to do tomorrow to be ready as a junior guide at the historic museum. It's going to be great."

Mom gave me a big hug. The image of me dressed in an orange jumpsuit suddenly changed to me as a pilgrim on Thanksgiving morning.

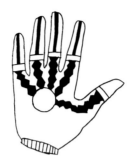

CHAPTER EIGHT
Don't Touch the Merchandise

I had one day to cram in as much information as I could about the House of Seven Gables into my size nine head. I propped myself up in bed with my laptop balanced on my stomach. I kept saying to myself that the house is one of only a few 17th century houses still standing in America. I repeated this fact like a mantra over and over in my head. Billy sat at the end of the bed staring at one of my old comic books.

"Do you think I can pull it off, Billy?"

Billy shrugged. "I don't know. I've never been to that old house. I don't really go anywhere."

"Well, I went there back at my old school in third grade, but I really didn't pay attention at all. All the kids were acting up, and the guide was so nervous someone would touch or even break something. I remember the ceilings were so low."

"I love jumping and trying to touch ceilings," Billy responded.

"You could probably touch these, Billy. Houses were built back then to conserve heat from a fireplace. Heat rises, so low ceilings retain the heat more efficiently."

I hoped some more of my fun facts in American history would keep kicking in before this job started. Mom was still mad at me for the stunts I played with Squirrel. She was watching me non-stop.

Mom even traded in my old phone and gave me a new one that had a tracking device permanently enabled and a parental lock engaged. She was following my every move. She could even tell when I was in the bathroom. It was like she was one of those drones hovering over the neighborhood having me under constant surveillance, always watching.

I put on some beige shorts and a matching beige shirt. I had a special pin labeled "trainee." It was mandatory I wear it on my shirt. I felt like I was one step below wearing an orange jumpsuit and picking up trash like a convict on the side of the highway. I shot up from my bed, and Billy was already gone. He never hung around for too long.

Getting my bike out from the storage unit in the apartment's basement was good for me to do. My nurse told me it was good exercise to have to carry it up the stairs and might be easier than running. I was a bit high in my blood sugar check this morning, so a ten-minute bike ride toward the ocean was good for me and should allow my blood sugar to drop a bit. Well, that was how it is supposed to work scientifically. It didn't always happen that way.

I pulled up in front of the Turner House, otherwise known as the House of Seven Gables. Mr. McGovern read us a portion of the book by the same name by this town's famous local author Nathaniel Hawthorne this year, but it went over a fifth grader's head like a paper airplane. Hawthorne's writing was from the 1800s and a bit hard to comprehend. I struggled at times to understand books even from *this* century. I parked my bike around the back of the house and locked it to a metal pole for safe keeping. I didn't want to blow it anymore with tsunami Mom, or at least not for a while until the storm I had created finally subsided.

I met my supervisor, Mandy. She oversaw my community service hours. As part of the deal with the police, I had to check in and out with her every day and get a signature. She was tall, lean, and slightly mean.

Her brown eyes sized me up and down like a Slinky. I kept adjusting my ranger hat and had a little bead of sweat forming while she x-rayed me.

"So, Zander. The boys in blue caught you," Mandy said while tossing a piece of gum into her mouth.

"Sort of. I messed up a bit this summer. I was just trying to help my mom out," I responded.

"Every ex-convict that has ever walked through here has a story, my tall friend. You did the crime, now you will have to clean the grime," she said with a smirk. "With me."

"It wasn't really a crime. More like a misunderstanding."

Mandy walked close enough to see the sweat on my forehead. I had to step back, so my ranger hat would not bump into her.

"Crime, misunderstanding. Different points of view. It's all the same to me, Xavier."

"It's Zander."

"Listen, Xavier, you mess up with me, and you will be cleaning the toilets in this place. We have almost 500 guests a day visiting an over 300-year-old house. Do you know what 500 visitors a day can do to a toilet? Do you have any idea?"

"I really don't. I really don't want to know," I stammered.

"You will become an expert in waste management if you ever slip up with me, tall little man. You really messed up this summer, and this job is going to put you back on the straight and slim."

"Understood."

"You better understand. Be here on time, stay focused, and head home. Any more mess-ups and you won't be returning to that fancy private school of yours. You might be at a school for troubled boys. It's the type of place where you don't bring your blue blankie to bed after lights out. Understood?"

Was she psychic? How did she know about my blue blanket? I did not enjoy her description of a potential future. I had no friends here and no distractions to get me in trouble. No one even knew I would be here for a month serving my hours.

Mandy walked me through the rooms of the house. It was converted into a museum in the early 1900s after being built in the late 1600s. The dark wood covered house was famous for having seven gables jutting out from the top floor and onto the roof. Mandy took me into one of the family rooms with a central fireplace.

"Notice anything unusual in this room, trainee?" she asked.

I examined the room. I was just getting a grasp of what life was like in the 1850s.

"It has old pots in the fireplace?" I stabbed at the air for an answer.

"Of course, it has pots in the hearth! How do you think people boiled water and ate? Do you see many chairs in this room?"

I saw one long bench by the eating table. "Just that one."

"Exactly. A bench to eat. Do you see any comfortable chairs or rocking chairs? Any place for you to just relax after doing some work?" she asked.

"I don't. Were they all destroyed?"

"No, they weren't destroyed. People back in this time did not have resting chairs or rocking chairs. There was no time to sit down. When you were done with your work you ate or slept. When you finished one job, you moved on to the next. There was no sitting and relaxing in a chair."

"Oh," I said.

Mandy popped another piece of gum in her mouth and seemed to become even more exasperated with me.

"You kids, always online, always lounging around. Stand up straight and get to work!"

Mandy marched me back to the foyer to help with my first tour group.

I was introduced to a recent high school graduate named Tim. He was very friendly and gave me tips all day.

"Zander don't worry about crazy Mandy. She's intense. Too intense for her own good. Stick with me. Be polite, try to answer questions, and make sure your visitors come away with at least two facts learned. Make it worth their time. Especially the little ones. This town has beaches, an arcade, and a fishing pier just down the street. Don't you think most kids want to be there on a summer day instead of touring an old house with absolutely no video games or air conditioning?"

I nodded affirmatively and assisted tour guide Tim all day. Touring groups started on the hour, and this gave me one hour off for lunch. I had to assist five groups per day. The first group moved through the house with no issues, and I became slightly bored the second and third time around when I heard Tim's exact speech again. I was starting to get a sense of how my favorite teacher, Mr. McGovern's, teaching life was when he had to say the same thing multiple times a day and year after year. Tim was doing a good job making each tour seem fresh and new when I knew he had been giving the same speech all summer.

I sat under the cool shade of an oak tree in front of the House of Seven Gables. Mom had packed me a low-carb protein shake, yogurt, an apple, celery sticks, carrots (just a few carbs), and a piece of chicken. I knew I had diabetes every second of the day, but I wanted a dripping chocolate donut, a milkshake, and a candy bar occasionally. I didn't care that my pancreas took a lifetime vacation, and I had to take a shot to my arm, my leg, my stomach or even my butt to eat all that tasty junk food.

I was chewing my cold rubbery chicken when I saw a vision come across the parking lot. It was hot as blazes out, and I had to wipe the sweat off from under my ranger hat. The vision materialized into the shape of a girl, and she was waving at me.

"Hey, Zander! I thought it was you!" said Cynthia Prowse.

Cynthia sat down next to me. Cynthia was the most amazing fifth grader. She was smart, talented, and very pretty. I was her partner in science class when we had to build the Eiffel Tower out of craft sticks. I barely said anything to her all year. She measured everything. Her mother even sent us photos of the actual tower because she was doing a book tour in Paris. Her mother was a published author, and her intelligence really trickled down to her daughter.

"What are you doing here?" I asked her.

"I thought I would bike down since my mom is in final preparations for the opening of a new section of the Yin Yu Tang house tomorrow. I was getting bored and wanted to come by for a tour."

I was scratching my head. "You wanted to come over here?"

She whacked me on the arm. "You know I am a history aficionado. And the gift shop has great candy. I haven't been there in months."

She nodded toward the house. Cynthia reached into my sandwich bag and stole a few carrot sticks.

"My mom is part of the big ceremony tomorrow at the museum with the new exhibit."

"The Win Yu Tang house?"

"Yin Yu Tang House. You remember my family is directly related to it?" She nudged me.

"Yeah, the whole school knows that, Cynthia. You tell everyone every five seconds."

Cynthia belly laughed.

"I'm sorry for that. I've settled down now. I've matured." She raised her eyebrow to me.

"Really? So, have I. Take a gander at me, a park ranger!" I pointed to the glimmering medal on my chest.

"Pretty fancy. You haven't been into any trouble this summer? It's been all chill and quiet?"

"Quiet as a mouse," I said.

"What about that troublemaking friend of yours? You used to mention him during lunch, what was his name? Rabbit? Chipmunk?"

"Squirrel. He's around. He's helping to clean up a highway this week."

"Really— 'helping' is an interesting choice of words."

I could have chatted with Cynthia all day, but I had a few more afternoon tours, and Cynthia was joining my next one.

Cynthia wrote down facts that Tim said during the tour into her notebook. I kept trying to peek over to see what she was writing, but she turned her shoulder away from me and shook her head. She really did want to be a writer like her mother. Cynthia was actually enjoying herself as she learned about life in the 1800s.

I spent most of my time herding kids and stragglers from room to room and making sure people did not step past any of the ropes or touch the beds and furniture. I had one peculiar gentleman under my watchful eyes the entire tour. His nametag read "Bruce," and he was wearing a Batman themed t-shirt straining to hold his girth. He was a bit too preoccupied videotaping every room and was not too mindful of his surroundings. In more than one room, I had to make sure he did not bump into a lamp or lean into a glass cabinet.

"You like my gear, kid?" said Bruce.

I nodded yes and turned to him.

"Good, because you are live streaming on my YouTube channel right now."

Bruce turned and had replaced his handheld camera with a small camera mounted directly on his glasses. He flipped a switch and a spotlight blasted across my face like the bat signal. Tim covered his eyes at the front of the line and motioned the group to keep moving forward.

"Talk to my subscribers, tour guide Zander. I have over one million people following me every day."

Bruce turned his head and scanned the whole room.

"Follow you doing what?" I asked.

"You haven't heard of Bruce TV? Where have you been living? In a cave?"

"With my mom, and often we don't get a very good internet signal in our apartment."

"I live stream almost all my daily activities except the personal things. I tour around Salem and the Boston area covering topics of interest both big and small. I've streamed everything—from kids doing trick shots, to ninja cats, to llamas eating peanut butter. My followers will watch anything I post. Check these out."

Bruce reached into his backpack and pulled out two gloves. He carefully slipped them on and pressed a small power button on the wrist of each hand.

"You thought the goggles were great. These are pure multisensory virtual reality. It transmits thousands of bits of information with everything I touch," Bruce said.

He reached out and grabbed my arm.

"Hey!" I moved away from him.

"Just a demonstration, my friend. I quickly swiped your arm, and now the sensors in the fingertips of my gloves are relaying to Bruce TV who you are and all your information. My followers will determine if you are worthy enough to investigate further. The gloves could also tell me all your vitals such as height, weight—oh, what is this?"

Bruce was peering intently into his goggles.

"You are a diabetic?"

"I have diabetes. How did you know that?"

"The gloves know all."

"The gloves and their owner don't know much about privacy, do they?" said Cynthia.

"These gloves can read the fluctuations in your blood sugar. It is a 350 right now. Are you feeling loopy or angry?"

I glared at the oversized robotic man, and I was furious. I couldn't believe his technology could read my blood sugar. This would save me the time of stabbing my fingers six times a day. I examined my fingers riddled with tiny black and blue bruises.

"How much do they cost?" I asked.

"Each glove is $15,000," said Bruce.

I gulped hard. Bruce scanned me with his gloves. "You should really get an insulin pump, or a glucose monitor my friend. It will help you manage your blood sugar."

I was now hearing advice from a cyborg? I just nodded. I wanted him to stop talking since my mother and every one of my doctors had been trying to get me on a pump for years. If I went on a pump that meant I'd always have to SEE my diabetes. It would be attached to me and a constant reminder of this disease.

"So be careful around me, kids," Bruce announced. "I am an expensive machine-man."

Bruce wandered into the next room, and I followed him. Museum guide Tim finished each tour by visiting the main kitchen area. He stopped by the fireplace.

"Gather around, everyone. Here is the central meeting place for family life in the 17th and 18th centuries. This room contained the house's central fireplace with pots hanging over it. A large kitchen table and chairs were placed on the outskirts of the room. When this house was turned into a museum in the early 1900s, the owners did not need all six of the house's fireplaces to work. Could someone open up that broom closet please?"

I smiled because this was the part every visitor waited for. A small boy opened the door to find stairs.

"Cool, a secret staircase!" The boy peeked his head in.

Tim smiled. "The owners hollowed out a giant chimney and installed a secret staircase all the way up to the bedrooms. The stairs spiral up inside the chimney all the way to the top floor. Let's go up there before we finish in the gift shop."

Tim told the group to be careful and hold the railing as they twisted up the staircase. The excitement was almost palpable. Tim led the line with the small children going first. I stood at the end to make sure everyone had cleared the kitchen. I didn't want anyone sneaking around the house. Bruce turned on his gloves and rubbed them against the uneven brick walls. He stepped slowly.

"What are you doing?" I asked.

"I am taking a sensory inventory for my followers." He was rubbing his hands over the bricks and the railing. "The gloves are taking in all the information, and my followers can see when the bricks were made, what the material is made out of, and hundreds of other facts."

"Fascinating," I mumbled.

As we reached the top of the stairs, a small boy at the front of the line tripped on a step and Cynthia reached out to grab him. He fell back for a second and bumped into Bruce. Bruce was too busy glove scanning to see the boy bump him in the stomach. Bruce lurched back. I saw his larger-than-life sweaty backside come toward me with the open spiral staircase of darkness behind me. I did not want to go backward at all. I threw my hands out to stop Bruce but primarily to keep myself from falling to my doom. Bruce finally snapped out of his virtual reality and into our reality while he was falling back. He threw his hands out against the pitted bricks of the hollowed-out chimney. He slid his hands back and slammed them into pieces of iron sticking out.

"Stop pushing me! Watch out for my gloves!" Bruce yelled.

I heard this as I pressed him forward with all my strength. Bruce's weight was pushing more and more against me. I felt my fingers sliding into the damp folds of his back fat. It was at that moment I heard the ripping sound of fabric.

"No, no!"

Tim was waiting with the group, and Cynthia watched as Bruce slowly walked up the stairs and pulled off his goggles. I walked into the bedroom last and rubbed my hands together. I could feel the aching of my wrists from pushing Bruce forward.

Bruce held his hands out to me and Cynthia.

"What have you done?" he asked angrily.

"Zander didn't do anything. It was an accident. A boy tripped, and Zander stopped you from falling down those spiral stairs and cracking your head open," Cynthia responded.

"Lies, this boy pushed me, and look what happened," Bruce said.

He was pointing directly at me. His bare skin was exposed through a large tear in each glove. He slowly pulled them off and held them gently like a newborn puppy.

"They are useless now and beyond repair. Do you know how much these costs?" Bruce was getting angrier in his tone.

"Yes, you told everyone $30,000 multiple times during the tour. Hopefully you have insurance?" Cynthia asked.

"I'm not sure, but this kid is going to pay for them." Bruce pointed directly at me.

I was shaking my head. "I don't have that kind of money," I said. "I don't even have $300."

Cynthia stepped between me and Bruce. "He's not going to pay for it mister. It was an accident."

Tim walked over. "It was an accident, and we can talk to the director in the gift shop as to what the policy is when someone has an accident."

Bruce cradled his shredded gloves. "This was not an accident. This was intentional."

Cynthia rolled her eyes.

"You are going to pay. I swear," Bruce said.

"Are you kidding me? What are you going to do? Put a hex on him? Please." Cynthia nudged me to the back of the bedroom toward the sign that pointed to the gift shop.

"If this doesn't get settled, I will curse you, my diabetic friend, for the rest of your life!" he shouted across the room.

Great. I was now going to be cursed by a technology-nut who has a million online followers. He'd post the whole encounter, and I'd be the laughing stock of sixth grade in September. I could barely make enough money this summer, the police were tracking me on this job, and now the whole online world would know my failures.

I sat on a long bench in the gift shop and peeled my nametag off my shirt. I wiped the sweat from my head and reached in my pocket for a bag of peanuts. Peanuts are high protein, low carb, and I didn't inject to have this quick snack.

Cynthia sat down next to me. She reached into her gift bag and pulled out a stuffed doll version of the author Nathaniel Hawthorne. She snuggled him into my face.

"Brighten up, Zander. I am sure the adults will work it out. You were helping. I saw you save him."

"It was really just a big push."

"It was a save. It was pretty cool."

Cynthia made the little stuffed author Nathaniel dance across my folded arms.

"So, Zander, are you working Saturday?" Cynthia asked.

"Surprisingly, I am actually free."

"Do you want to come to the museum opening with me? There is a big ribbon cutting ceremony, and my Mom said I could bring a friend."

"Sounds fun."

"Be there at noon and leave the cargo shorts at home. It's going to be slightly fancy."

I watched Cynthia head out the door, and I waved goodbye to her. This afternoon was the most I had ever said to her even after a whole school year and many projects together. Was it a date? I never had a date before. I chomped on my peanuts and turned my attention back to the front desk where Bruce was filling out forms and staring at me menacingly. I gulped the dry peanuts down my throat.

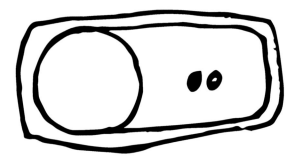

CHAPTER NINE
Tang's Trouble

I woke up the next morning to see five texts from my Dad, or Trevor, as I started calling him after he left us. Squirrel was right about Trevor getting a gig as an undead zombie. I still could not believe I spotted an action figure of him at the comic store. I was sure some boys would love to have an action figure of their father. My dad's figure had his head partially detached, a shovel through his chest and blood coming out of his eyes. I would settle on him being a decent dad bobblehead instead. It will be three years this Christmas since he skipped town. He said he always had unfinished business and was an underachiever. Trevor tried to talk to me then like an adult when I was a third grader. I didn't understand what he was saying, but I did understand when he didn't come back.

My mom was working nonstop during that time. I felt terrible, and I was wetting the bed. Talk about embarrassing. Mom thought it was a case of stress—of them fighting and arguing—but I wasn't so sure. I felt awful, and finally, Mom took me to her hospital. I gave her a cup filled with my urine, and she dipped a special stick into it. She watched as the stick changed color, and her face portrayed devastation. I had traces of protein in my pee, and the sugar level in my blood was enough to keep me in the hospital for days.

I walked out by the end of the week with a bag full of needles, ridiculous amounts of insulin to take, and my head overloaded with the fact that I had to take shots with all my food. Mom and I walked all the way home that day since she had to sell the car. Dad was nowhere to be found.

I stared at his name on the phone and retyped the "Dad" contact to now read "Trevor." I clicked on it and it said, "I'll be back." The second one said, "See you soon." I deleted the next three. I guess he was coming back, but I would only believe it when he was standing in front of me. He said that when I was finishing third grade, then again in fourth grade, and now that I was about to enter sixth grade. Talk about not keeping your promises, Trevor.

I rolled myself out of bed to hear the TV. Billy was sitting in front of it watching cartoons. I checked my blood sugar. It was a lowly 50. I had a few beads a sweat on my head and knew I was getting lower. If I didn't eat soon, I was going to be on the floor passed out, and Billy would not be any help. He didn't even know how to use a phone. I poured myself a huge bowl of Cap'n Crunch and decided to not inject myself with any insulin. I was fading fast and the cereal would fill me up. I knew I should be having some juice to bring me up and then later take my insulin with the cereal, but I was just too hungry and way too impatient. I was going to have an unhealthy high blood sugar number, but this plan would allow me to not have to prick my finger and ooze blood in front of Cynthia. There was nothing more embarrassing than having to do all my finger pricking and blood checking in front of other people. My mom kept telling me there was nothing wrong about doing this in public, but I just didn't like to have strangers stare at me. And now, I'd never forget that security guard yelling at me at the hotel.

I crunched, crunched, and crunched the cereal until the spoon banged against the bottom of the bowl. Mom didn't like dirty dishes, so I washed it right away.

"Bye, Billy. I am going out for the day! See you tonight!" Billy didn't respond. He just rocked in his chair, watching cartoons. He acted more and more depressed this summer. I really had not spent any time with him.

I was about to reach for my steadfast cargo shorts when I remembered Cynthia's only note about getting semi-fancily dressed. I searched my cluttered bedroom wall to see what I wore for my fifth-grade classroom picture and grabbed the same outfit: dress pants and a short sleeve collared shirt. I pulled the pants up, and the waist fit just fine. I was showing off too much of my ankles. I put on a pair of socks to match the beige pants and hide the fact I had outgrown the pants. I grabbed the smallest backpack I had and tossed in my water bottle, walnuts, insulin kit, meter, and some Skittles. Mom didn't like me eating the candy, but it was the best way to raise my blood sugar quickly when I was feeling the lows. I really didn't want to be snacking on edamame beans or whatever kale or ginger snaps she was trying to force down my throat from a farm to table kick she was on. It was more like a farm to trash can when I saw all the healthy items come home. Also, those types of snacks would not help my lows quickly.

The Peabody Essex Museum was a shorter walk from my house than my current job at the House of Seven Gables. It was built as a museum to celebrate Salem's maritime history, and the town's connection to its sea trading past in Europe and Asia. Years ago, the museum bought a two-story house that was built in the 1700s in China. After the old house was purchased, it was taken apart brick-by-brick, nail-by-nail, and then reassembled as an addition to this Salem museum thousands of miles away. I could not believe that a house could be taken apart, put into hundreds of crates, and then put back together perfectly in another country. It was tough enough for me to assemble one Lego set.

Cynthia was waiting for me at the front of the Yin Yu Tang house. I walked through the museum's lobby to see her waving me over. Her dimpled smile demonstrated she was happy to see me.

"You remembered about the no cargo shorts," she said. I politely nodded. "You clean up well, Zander. Dad, this is Zander from my class at Flowing Meadows."

I reached over to shake her father's hand.

"Pleasure to meet a classmate of Cynthia's. You can call me Tom."

Tom waved our group toward the door and into the house.

"The museum is reopening one of the rooms in the Yin Yu Tang house today, Zander. It's a big deal. We can trace our family's heritage back many generations in this house. It was built in the 1700s in Eastern China and held generations and generations of the Huang family members until the 1950s," said Cynthia.

"Then, what happened?" I asked.

"My dad's family had already moved to America in the early 1900s, and all other cousins and uncles were gone from the house. It fell into shambles until the museum bought it around 2000."

Cynthia opened the wooden door of the house and a small group of people entered the ground floor. It was a two-story building with an opening in the room that allowed light to fall into the central courtyard. I could only compare it to a motel with rooms on the outside walls and a shallow pool filled with green water in the middle.

"I can't believe it was moved here brick-by-brick, Cynthia."

"It's pretty unbelievable. My dad has been ridiculously active with the museum to help renovate each room. This is a big deal to have another room out of the twenty rooms fully restored to a specific time period. Dad was instrumental in finishing this project. I can tell how excited he is. He doesn't really smile that often. What does your dad do again, Zander?"

"It's a little different lifestyle choice. He preys upon unsuspecting humans and eats their brains. He doesn't discriminate in his eating selection. A brain is a brain."

Cynthia gave me a quizzical eyebrow raise. I was about to tell her what that smart aleck response meant when her dad spoke.

"Here is the Yin Yu Tang House's latest room. It will be open to the public this afternoon. This house sheltered members of my family for over 200 years until the 1950s. This bedroom is now a complete representation of what it was like for one of the last members of my family to stay here in 1951. The museum has faithfully recreated the room based off of the time period, family letters, photographs, and stories from grandparents. The writing desk is original to the room and was tracked down a few years ago."

I went over to put my hand on it, and Cynthia politely pulled me back and whispered about a no touching policy in the house.

"At least wait until the tour goes back down the stairs," she said.

Tom continued his tour. "Young adults in China were often intended to be married or already married by the age of fourteen. It was completely common to start families that young."

I turned my head to Cynthia, and her eyes bugged out. I couldn't believe that.

"Young families were starting young and always planning ahead to not get into any trouble."

Cynthia turned to me. "Well, Mr. Burke, do you plan ahead? Are you marrying at 14?"

"I don't even plan my next meal. It's probably what makes me not very good with my diabetes. I can't imagine getting married so young and being with that person for the rest of my life."

"If you find the right person, age shouldn't really matter," she whispered.

My head was spinning. I didn't understand what she was saying. I wasn't sure if she was thinking of marrying me or if I was getting a diabetic low. Cynthia was staring at the family photos on the wall when I pointed to a wooden barrel next to the bed that had a small opening at the top.

"What is this, Cynthia? Is this for dirty laundry?"

"It is called a child minder."

I raised my eyebrows, not understanding.

"Remember my dad said Chinese families were always planning ahead? When the couple had a baby, they would put the baby in this."

Cynthia grabbed a pillow from the bed, turned it on its side and gently slid it halfway down into the opening of the wooden vase.

"The baby sits straight up, can't fall through, can do all the kicking he or she wants and more importantly can't get into any trouble."

"That's pretty ingenious. An old-fashioned portable baby crib."

The group headed back to the hallway overlooking the courtyard. I could feel a breeze coming in from the open roof. A man in the back of the group lowered his phone from his face to see me.

"Hey, I know you," he said. He came over to me to shake my hand. "We met a little while back. I'm Ernie Reynolds, the movie producer."

I told Cynthia that I had met Ernie at the hotel while he was putting up casting signs for the upcoming zombie movie that he would film in Salem. I didn't tell Cynthia the part that I had met the producer just before I landed in jail.

"It's finally happening. We have all the locations. In less than two weeks we will shoot here for almost a month."

"Shooting what?" Cynthia asked.

"The Witches Apocalypse. It's going to be epic. Tortured souls from the 17th century return to seek revenge on present day townspeople. We are shooting all over Salem to keep it authentic. We have already shot most of the film in Canada and will film the final battle scenes here."

Ernie glanced down at his phone and scrolled through his texts. I pulled my phone out to see the text from my dad that said, "I'll be back." Now I know what that meant. He was a top zombie in Hollywood. He even had his own action figure. I bet he was coming back for these scenes. I first tried phone calls, then hand-written letters in cursive, and my last attempts were rudimentary third grade emails.

Nothing was successful in bringing him back to Mom and me. It took a zombie apocalypse to finally bring my father back home.

Ernie kept staring at his phone.

"This guy keeps bugging me. He can't take a hint when I don't call him back. He started out as lead extra, and now he has a line or two of dialogue. He's actually just grunting and moaning."

"Is that a big deal?" I asked.

"Huge, because now it's a great payday for him even if he utters one word. It doesn't even have to be a coherent word or in English. In his case, he mumbles a word or two since he's a zombie. I will give it to him that he is top notch as a zombie. He is one of the best zombies in Hollywood right now."

Ernie's phone vibrated.

"It's him calling again! I can't believe it!"

Ernie showed us the phone. I read the caller identification as "Trevor."

I started to feel lightheaded.

"I would block him if only I knew how to on this new phone."

I felt the sweat tingling on my forehead. My feet wobbled. Ernie finally answered his phone.

"Hello, this is Ernie. Yes, Trevor I received all your texts. You MAY have another line or zombie groan. It counts as the same thing as English, and you'll be paid. I know that will change the contract. Talk to my assistant the day before shooting starts in Salem. He will work out all the details. Don't worry, I said you will be compensated. You know how to get to Salem, Massachusetts, right?"

Ernie was nodding and rolling his eyes at me.

"I'm actually here scouting a location in a Salem museum. I'm on a tour with a small group in part of a Chinese house. Maybe it will be destroyed by the zombies next month during the apocalypse. The director and I are still figuring it out. No, no. I'm with a tour. I am with a middle schooler named Zander. I think he will be in the production next month if he's not too busy."

Ernie winked at me.

"He could be one of our final survivors and be in the big explosion scene. The top secret one."

Ernie smiled at me and then pressed his ear to his phone.

"Your son is named Zander, and he's from Salem? What a coincidence! This boy is almost my height, tall, short brown hair. He could start shaving soon. Ah, adolescence. What's that? He's probably your son? You don't say. Small world."

Ernie pulled the phone away from his ear.

"Is this nutcracker really your dad? He doesn't even know what you look like. I don't get it."

Ernie brought the phone back to his ear.

"Okay, but I have to wrap this up. I'll see you soon. Talk to my assistant again, he will work out your payment."

Ernie pulled the phone away from his ear and turned the screen to get closer and closer to me. Sweat was pouring down my face. I saw the name "Trevor" get larger and larger. The caller ID showed my zombified Dad with his head surprisingly attached to his body. The phone and the zombie descended upon me.

"He wants to talk to you. Can you make it quick? I have to check out another location."

The phone was almost to my ear. I could hear the faint sound of my father saying, "Hello?" I leaned all my bodyweight into Cynthia and knocked her over. My legs gave way as my body hit the end of the authentic 1951 Zhen Zhi imported bedframe. I rolled and landed my bottom directly into the child minder at the end of the bed.

Cynthia told me this much later. I blacked out when the image of zombie Dad and his voice rang in my head.

I woke up in a very comfortable bed with an IV attached to my right arm, a heartbeat monitor on my left index finger, and a very uncomfortable lower back.

"Good evening, sleepy head."

I turned to see Mom sitting in a chair next to my bed. She looked at me intently while holding a large textbook and highlighters in her lap.

"You passed out," she said.

"I guessed that judging by the situation."

"What do you remember?" she whispered.

"I was talking to Cynthia and became dizzy. It wasn't like my typical diabetes dizzy low feeling. I had no warning this time. I knew I had to lie down. Get on the ground, so I wouldn't hurt myself. I didn't even have time to get my snack from my backpack."

"You were lucky, Zander. There were a bunch of people around you at the museum. The paramedics came and gave you an emergency glucose shot. You were not unresponsive for very long."

"Unresponsive?" I said. I knew that term was very bad in the medical world and a very troubling word in the diabetes community.

"The EMT brought you here, and here we are—many hours later."

"I guess that was pretty serious, Mom."

"I know it was. You do remember that your grandfather, my father, died from complications from this disease. I know I don't talk about him enough, and he certainly never liked to talk about his diabetes. He mostly hid it from everyone. He would be amazed at the advances in medicine now available to you."

"What are you talking about?" I responded.

My mom held a small silver device about the size of a walnut in her palm. I sat up in bed.

"Is that what I think it is, Mom?"

"It is. It's a CGM or a continuous glucose monitor. It tests your glucose level every five minutes and sends the number wirelessly to your phone...and more importantly, to mine."

"It's a modern-day child minder! A tracker for me. I told you I don't want one."

"I watched you sleep for the past few hours Zander. Every doctor that came in here asked me why you are not on this little device. I've been holding it the whole time, and each doctor said it should be on you doing its job. Your life was in danger. You were not monitoring your glucose levels well enough. You probably had not checked all day today. This is serious."

Mom reached over from her chair and grabbed my hands.

"This device will give us better information, so you don't get into trouble again. You are coming up on almost three years with this disease. You are entering full-blown hormonal adolescence, and your numbers are going crazy. This device will give us quite a bit of information to keep you healthy and safe. How many situations have you had this summer? This device will give a warning if you are low, so you don't end up passed out somewhere or back in this hospital bed." Mom was exasperated.

"A warning?" I said.

Mom pointed to the light on the device. "It will go from a functioning solid green to yellow and finally an alarm will go off with the red light. It means if you are under 50, you should have a snack quickly to raise your blood sugar."

"I know what a 50 means, Mom. Is it a comforting and soothing alarm?" I asked, sarcastically.

Mom's nostrils flared. I crossed my arms. I was not happy. This day started out perfectly well. This morning I was hanging out with Cynthia, and by the evening I was getting the real hard sell on technology that I did not want attached to my body. I had barely talked to Cynthia all year, and I finally spent the entire day with her. We got along great during the tour, and my stupid diabetes ruined the whole event. She'll never talk to a freak like me again.

I turned away from Mom and stared at the wall.

"I know you are angry, Zander. You didn't ask for this disease. It probably has taken away much more than it has given you."

"Mom, do you know the last image I saw before I blacked out?"

"Hopefully, your sweet mother?"

"No, it was Zombie Dad."

Mom tilted her head quizzically. "Zombie Dad?"

"It was Dad, or Zombie Dad now because I guess he's a really good zombie actor in Los Angeles. He was calling me, and then I passed out. I am not sure if it was a coincidence or the cause."

Mom crossed her arms. She pushed a long breath through her nostrils.

"Did you talk to him?"

"No, but he's been bugging the movie producer for a month. I guess he's part of the movie."

"The zombie movie that's filming all over town?"

Mom shook her head.

"He'll be here. He's been trying to call me. He was talking to the producer, and then the producer figured out I was his son. The whole situation is really confusing."

"It typically is when your father is involved. Figures, after all these years, he has returned only for this movie. He missed everything, and now he's going to waltz back in here on the red carpet."

"Zombies don't really waltz, Mom. They sort of lurch."

"Well, Zander. Your father's return after all these years makes our final conversation of the night so much easier now."

Mom reached forward and handed me a card. It read, "Dr. Teresa Storm, Adolescent Psychologist." I put the card down on my lap.

"She's different than your old therapist. She works with older kids, and she works out of her house. I thought a new therapist would be more successful this time. Dr. Storm is doing me a big favor. She agreed to see you for the rest of the summer. Things have not been going well. Your poor decision-making, the lying to me about the job situation, an emergency hospital visit, and now your father returning. It's a set-up for disaster. You need someone to talk to. I understand you are getting older and that person to talk to is not always going to be me. We have to get a better handle on your life."

Mom put the CGM device back in its box and placed it on a table. At the doorway, little Billy stood with his arms crossed. He glared at me and did not look happy.

"I guess you're right, Mom. I probably do need someone to talk to."

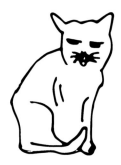

CHAPTER TEN
Mr. Cuddles

I had finally done it. I was in the nut house. This place must've been filled with crazy squirrels fighting over the last nut before winter. I had the card for the shrink, Dr. Teresa, and made the call. Mom always made me make the calls concerning my health. She said it taught me good phone etiquette and how-to self-advocate. I was cleared to leave the hospital and return to my job at the House of Seven Gables. I had to go back there, or I would be in trouble for leaving and in even bigger trouble with the local police. Mom made sure the shrink session was set up and that I would be there. I think she had been overusing the tracking option on my phone. She could find my location anytime, anywhere. There was no escape.

    I thought I was in the wrong part of town when I biked past my job at the House of Seven Gables and kept peddling toward the Atlantic Ocean. I peddled past the arcade, a creepy fortune-teller, and the wafting odors of popcorn, pizza, and Chinese food. My phone directed me to ride to the end of amusement park row, take a sharp right when I saw a long pier, and turn onto Beach Avenue. I didn't see any doctor's offices, only old houses overlooking the Atlantic Ocean and waves crashing against huge rocks.

I pulled up to the last house on Beach Avenue. The house was two stories tall with weathered gray shingles and black shutters. I locked my bike up against the mailbox post. The address on the business card matched the "33" on the mailbox.

"This must be the place."

I took the first step onto her porch, and the wood let out a huge creak. It felt like any foot pressure was going to send me through the steps in an instant. The creaking became louder with each rising step as I finally reached her front door. My finger was about to hit her doorbell when I heard…

"Come in, Zander,"

I opened the screen door and tiptoed inside. Dr. Teresa Storm whisked into the room. She was wearing a black robe or a cape. I could not really tell what it was. She had white hair with a startling black streak running down it. She was also wearing sunglasses, even though the room was extremely dark.

"Excuse me for my rudeness with the glasses. I just had my eyes dilated, and they are highly sensitive to light. Would you like some tea?"

"No, thanks."

I was visibly nervous standing in her foyer area. I saw mirrors, family pictures, and many lit candles. It smelled like one of those candle stores at the mall that I never wanted to enter. I heard a creak on the stairs and turned back to see Billy peeking in the screen door.

"Head on into my study in the next room and make yourself comfortable. I'm just getting my tea ready for our session."

I saw Billy put his hand on the screen door.

"Billy, you need to stay outside," I whispered loudly.

Billy let go of the doorknob and gave me a scowl. Dr. Storm turned toward me.

"Did you ask me something, Zander?"

"No, ma'am. Just clearing my throat," I said. I hope she had not heard that. It would just add to the list of my already lengthy physical and mental ailments. After hearing the screen door bang a few times, I took a seat on her extremely comfortable sofa. I felt a rubbing on my legs and saw a cat massaging itself against me. Dr. Storm walked in with her black dress flowing behind her. I couldn't tell what it was, but I was still fascinated by it. It was like she was floating across the floor. Her big bug sunglasses only added to the mystery.

"Mr. Cuddles, scram." She stomped her foot down, and the cat went running out of the room.

"Yes, the name is Mr. Cuddles. I found the cat as a stray with only a tag stating "Mr. Cuddles." I then had the veterinarian examine the cat's underside, and we couldn't tell if it was a boy or girl. The cat is now the gender-neutral Mr. Cuddles. They're real sweet but get into oodles of trouble."

Mr. Cuddles scuttled out of the room. Dr. Storm offered me tea or water. I chose the water. I took a big gulp, and I could see the doctor with the dark bug-eyed glasses turn her full attention to me. She locked in, and there was nowhere to run.

"So, Zander. I had your mother as a student last fall. I don't know how she manages her job, night classes, and single parenting. She will be a great nurse one day. She contacted me while you were sleeping in the hospital. I see you are almost twelve years old and have had type 1 diabetes for almost three years."

I nodded.

"Good," she said.

"There's nothing really good about diabetes, Dr. Storm."

"Oh, you misunderstood. I only meant good that I had my facts straight. It wasn't my opinion on the disease."

"I'm glad." I crossed my arms. I wasn't sure why I was giving Dr. Storm such a hard time. She was a bit quirky but seemed nice, and her house and paintings were keeping me thoroughly engaged.

"You manage this disease daily, almost hourly, and there is really no forgetting about it," she said.

"Exactly." I lifted the sleeve of my t-shirt to show the bruise on my left tricep.

"That's a nice bruise you have there, Zander. It looks like you must be left-handed and bolus or inject yourself into your right arm. Have you tried rotating your injection sites to not bruise so much?"

"I'm a creature of habit. I inject sometimes in the legs but never in the stomach or butt."

Dr. Storm took some notes down in her journal. I couldn't make out what she was writing.

"Zander, would you consider rotating your injection sites to break or at least bend some of your habits?"

I nodded. "Why not? I can try."

"Do you keep a journal to write down all your thoughts about your condition?" she asked.

"I wrote a little when I was first diagnosed. I was given a stack of coloring books, journals, daily food logs. It eventually all ended up all in a heaping pile in my room. My last therapist also asked me to write down some thoughts in a journal, and I just drew and scribbled."

"It might help you to jot down a few notes on some of your tough days. Sometimes a person gets too stuck inside one's own headspace and writing those thoughts down could help you get outside of your own head."

Dr. Storm surveyed the bookcase behind her and pulled out a small notebook. She flipped through it and handed it to me.

"Try this one. I feel this will be more successful than the last one. You are older now with so much more to say. Next time I see you maybe you can share a few thoughts you have written. If this doesn't work for you, some of my clients even type in some thoughts on their phones to share with me. I have evolved with the technology too."

I thought this might be a bit more likely to add a few pithy comments on my phone whenever something profane popped into my head.

"I don't want to spend our whole hour together talking about your diabetes. I bet you don't like it when that is all your mother asks you. She may ask you what your blood sugar number is the second you wake up or immediately when you come home from school. She asks about the disease first and the child later."

"I don't like that at all," I said.

"That's what I thought. You should not and will not be defined by your disease. You must be known and recognized by your words and your selfless actions, Zander. Not by your disability."

I never really connected diabetes to having an actual disability. Hearing Dr. Storm say that made me feel slightly better. I wanted people to know me for me and not for all the injections and finger pricking I had to do every day. I never wanted pity or sorrow from anyone.

"Your mom said something happened at the museum just as you were fainting. Can you tell me about that?"

Dr. Storm jotted down a few items in her notebook again. I really wanted to see what she was writing.

"I was not feeling so hot and getting a little dizzy when I was standing in the room with Cynthia at the Chinese house. I was talking to a producer named Ernie. He's producing a zombie movie here in Salem. He was having a heated chat with some nut job on the phone, and then Ernie put it together. The nut on the phone was related to this nut, me."

"How so?" she asked.

"The crazy crackpot was my disappearing dad. Producer Ernie showed me the phone, and I saw Zombie Dad. I will spare you the unnecessary questions and tell you that my father is now a top zombie actor in Hollywood. I saw the zombie face on the caller ID, heard his voice, and then blacked out."

"You had a physical and emotional reaction to seeing and hearing your father for the first time in almost three years."

"Well, I heard him but only saw Zombie Dad. Come to think of it, it's the only version of my dad I have seen since he left. I saw him on TV, and I saw an action figure of him as a zombie."

"So, Zander, Zombie Dad is the only version that you know of your dad since he left. Did you talk to anyone about it?"

"Mom asked me how I was feeling. She did quite a bit at first when he left us. When I was diagnosed with diabetes, I thought he would come home or call. He didn't. Mom slowly stopped talking about him. She worked more and more to keep up with the growing bills. I talked to Billy—"

I gasped after I said his name. Now she'd know I really am a nut.

"Who's Billy?" she asked.

I could not believe I said his name out loud. I am positive I have never said his name to anyone. Not even Squirrel. First the fact that my dad's coming home, then the hospital visit, and now my secret was blown about Billy. I heard the screen door bang on the porch. I bet Billy was still mad at me and slamming it to get my attention.

I took in a deep breath and exhaled slowly through my nose.

"Billy is my brother."

Dr. Storm reviewed her notes, and then flipped through a manila folder.

"You won't find his name listed on any form," I said.

"Okay, Zander. Now I am thoroughly confused."

I heard the banging of the screen door again.

"Billy showed up when my mom and dad starting fighting. I mean really fighting, yelling, screaming. It was real nasty. He just sort of arrived. He watched TV with me. I talked to him. He would follow me to school and around town."

"Is he here in the room with us?"

"No, I think he's outside on the porch or should be there at least."

Dr. Storm put her notebook down, and I knew she was going to ask me the question that I had been dreading since Billy showed up years ago. The banging grew louder.

"Zander. Is he really on the porch?"

I waited to answer her. I knew that what I was going to say would alter my situation. I needed things to change since whatever decisions I had been making were not the right decisions.

"He's my imaginary brother."

She stared politely at me for a while. It was a non-judgmental stare, and it gave me enough time to reach over to her coffee table and take a large gulp from a small water bottle.

"It's perfectly acceptable for young adults to have imaginary friends. Most tend to outgrow them in adolescence, and the friend simply fades away. The friend is considered irrelevant. Do you want Billy to fade away?"

"I think so. I haven't been very kind to him lately. I don't spend any time with him anymore, and I think he's mostly bored, angry, or both," I said.

"Maybe this is a perfect time for you to say your goodbye."

"Maybe," I whispered.

"Billy is a coping mechanism, Zander. He arrived at a time that was very turbulent for you. You needed someone to talk to, a friend, a brother in your case. He was the brother you never had or wished you had if your family unit stayed intact."

"I've been better this school year about meeting more people, and there will be some new classmates in September."

Dr. Storm glanced discretely at her watch. "It's about that time to wrap up our session for today. You have some work to do with Billy. We will get together at this same time in two weeks."

"Sounds good, my dad will be in town next week for the zombie movie filming. I might actually take some of that tea you offered next time."

Dr. Storm walked me to her front door, and I saw that the screen was slightly ajar. I hoped Billy hadn't left it open with all the banging during our session. I finally needed to say my goodbye to him. I walked out onto the porch to see my bike right where I left it against the mailbox.

"Oh no!" Dr. Storm yelled.

I saw Dr. Storm pointing frantically out toward the boulders at the end of her front yard. The boulder field formed a natural barrier between Dr. Storm's front lawn and the crashing waves of the ocean. She continued to point out toward one of the larger rocks. Perched on top of a boulder with striations across it sat Mr. Cuddles in all their feline glory. Mr. Cuddles was licking a front paw and staring back at us.

"They must have tiptoed out through the screen door. They're a really good house cat but not well behaved outdoors. That cat gets into so much trouble."

We both watched as the sporadic ocean waves crashed against her rock wall. The next wave hit Mr. Cuddles's rock with a wallop. I was hoping Mr. Cuddles would make it through the deluge. I closed my eyes as the wave hit Mr. Cuddles. I slowly opened them a second later to see a dripping wet Mr. Cuddles clinging for dear life and slowly sliding off the rock into the dark, ominous ocean.

"We need a rope or a net!" Dr. Storm yelled.

"Do you have any of those items?" I asked.

"No, I don't."

Mr. Cuddles continued sliding down the rock. They were trying to claw back up the rock unsuccessfully. I tossed my journal and phone on the grass, kicked off my sneakers, and ran across the lawn.

"What are you doing?" Dr. Storm yelled.

"I'm going to save your cat!" I gasped out as I ran across the lawn. I probably should have made the decision to just get my sneakers soaking wet. I hit my first batch of small jagged rocks near the water, and my feet sent pain signals immediately to my brain. The feet of diabetics are a bit oversensitive. This was not a good activity for me.

"Ouch, ouch, ouch."

Mr. Cuddles was very close to me now. The cat was just one more rock away when a wave hit me from the back and knocked me down. I slowly stood back up and wiped the stinging saltwater from my eyes. I could clearly see the rock, but Mr. Cuddles was not on it.

"Oh no, Zander look!" yelled Dr. Storm from the edge of her grass.

Mr. Cuddles was slowly floating out to sea with their front paws slapping at the water. Their brown and black hair weighed him down. A frantic feline face was bobbing up and down in the water.

"I don't think Mr. Cuddles can swim!" yelled Dr. Storm.

"You think?" I yelled back, but the waves muffled my response. I couldn't believe how much the water weighed down my shirt and shorts. I felt like I was swimming while wearing a winter blanket. The pockets of my shorts filled up with water and forced me under. Mr. Cuddles continued to bob up and down, but in just a few strokes I caught up to the wet beast.

"Take my hand, Mr. Cuddles."

I don't know why I said that since I didn't think cats understood English, and Mr. Cuddles certainly would not be able to give me an appropriate response. I reached Mr. Cuddles and gently pulled them to me by the base of their furry neck. I'd watched enough animal shows and remembered how mamas successfully picked up their young even with their teeth by grabbing the layer of fur between the shoulder blades.

I expected a warm embrace for this nautical rescue. With claws fully extended, Mr. Cuddles swiped viciously across my face. I turned away instinctively, but I felt a claw or two slash across my cheek. I pulled the ungrateful feline to my stomach, but I could feel it scratching away.

CLAW, CLAW.

I was going to miss one of my favorite t-shirts featuring an "Everything's Better with Bacon" tagline on it as Mr. Cuddles continued to rip it to shreds. I slowly walked out of the water. Dr. Storm was running toward us with a blanket.

I reached out for the blanket, and Dr. Storm quickly wrapped Mr. Cuddles in it. I was happy to give the frenzied wild beast back to her. Mr. Cuddles became quite docile and loving when the creature was back in the arms of its caretaker. Dr. Storm rocked the swashbuckling animal until they returned to a purring housecat. Dr. Storm put her face right up against Mr. Cuddles, and I feared for her eyes since my cheek was aching right now. Mr. Cuddles gave her a quick lick on the nose.

"You are a hero, Zander. You singlehandedly saved my family."

"It's no big deal," I said as I wiped away blood on my cheek.

"You were selfless, Zander. Thinking about something else and not worrying about the consequences. You need to come in and get bandaged up."

I waved my hand away. "I'm good, Dr. Storm. I don't think Mr. Cuddles wants to see me anymore. I'm just going to bike home for a hot shower and a little bit of antibiotic. It's been a bit too much excitement for one afternoon. The bike ride will help cool my nerves a bit."

Dr. Storm waved a final goodbye to me as I unlocked by bike. I watched her walk in while snuggling her baby feline. I turned around to see Billy standing in front of me.

"Did you have a good time with the doctor?" He was not happy.

"Yes, Billy, it was pretty good. I have to figure out how to make some more money and deal with Zombie Dad coming to town. I have made one decision through all this, and you are not going to like it."

Billy gazed up at me. "What is it?"

"It's time for you and me to say goodbye."

Billy kicked a few pebbles.

"Do you really mean it, Zander? No more talks? No more hanging out, comics, TV time?"

I stomped my sneakers only to see water drip out of them. My relationship with the fictional world wasn't really helping me anymore. I had to take a baby step forward.

"I really mean it, Billy. We need to leave each other. I just have too many things to do. I have too many eggs to juggle, and it's been scrambled for too long. I have to move ahead in my life, not backwards."

"Can we talk about this another day? I am really going to miss you. Can I ever come back and visit?"

"I don't think it works that way, Billy. It's not going to help me become unscrambled if we keep bumping into each other."

"Please, Zander. I like being with you," Billy said.

I shook my head no. I hopped on my bike and peddled past Billy and down the driveway. Before I turned off of Beach Avenue, I looked over my shoulder at Billy, and he was gone. The waves across the lawn gave a loud crash as Dr. Storm's screen door smashed against its frame. Maybe it was Mother Nature, maybe it was Billy. I would never see him again.

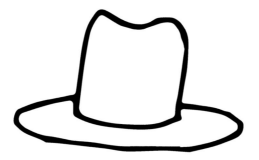

CHAPTER ELEVEN
The Zombies Arrive

"Will you get off that sofa and stop feeling sorry for yourself?" Squirrel whacked my stomach with today's paper. He showed me the headline that read "Feline Rescue."

"Look what the paper says. Have you even read the story?" Squirrel said.

I shook my head no.

"I will share the best part: 'Local youth Zander Burke raced into the turbulent water and pulled a helpless feline from the depths of the Atlantic Ocean. Mr. Burke sacrificed his safety to rescue a beloved family member. Both were uninjured after the nautical rescue.'"

"Okay, that's enough from that story, Squirrel. You shouldn't always believe what you read in the paper these days," I said.

"Why are you being so grumpy about this? This is fame and maybe some financial glory. You should be happy. Your mother is proud of you, and your therapist lady was the one who called the press about your heroic deed. The newspaper story pictures you as a local hero."

I sat up on the sofa. This was the first day without Billy. The little guy was around for almost three years, and I finally moved on. I forced it to happen. Billy really wasn't good for me anymore, but it still hurt. I needed to focus on reality and how to make my reality better with my mom and my diabetes.

It was quieter with Billy not around anymore. I had more time to myself and more time to think. I hoped for some quiet morning time until I woke up an hour ago to hear the TV. I walked out hoping not to see Billy. Sure enough, Billy wasn't there, but I did see Squirrel sitting on my sofa with the newspaper at his side and a large bowl of cereal on his lap.

"How did you even get in here?" I asked.

"Remember what I always say?" Squirrel responded.

"Squirrel knows all. Squirrel knows all," I said.

"I have known where your spare key is for years. Don't worry, I don't make a habit of coming in, eating your cereal, and watching TV while you sleep. That would be creepy."

Squirrel finished his cereal. I saw the article on the front page. It showed a picture of Mr. Cuddles wrapped in a blanket with his big soft eyes.

"I picked up a cat in the water. Period. The end."

Squirrel whacked me again with the paper.

"Are you kidding me? The newspaper headline should have read, 'Local boy risks life to save precious drowning family member.' I'm going to be your publicist from now on. You have too much going on. You need someone to sort and prioritize your life. I want to do this as your close and personal friend, Zander. Your life is much more exciting than mine. You have had police problems, situations at two local museums, driving well under the allowable age. We almost had a huge fight with a man-bun hipster while holding baseball bats, oh, and don't forget your possible movie role? See, you'll need an agent anyway. These situations don't happen to anyone but you. What about that YouTube virtual reality nut Bruce who is still foaming at the mouth and wants to sue you? I advise you not to read any of his online comments about what happened at the House of Seven Gables museum. Some posts are quite disturbing and highly inappropriate. And just when I thought things were getting quiet with you, BAM, a nautical feline rescue."

I rolled my eyes and tried to dismiss Squirrel's ranting.

"Listen buddy, anything next on your schedule needs to go through me. AND if there is money involved, I will gladly take a petty amount of ten percent as my commission. I'm just trying to make life easier for you, buddy." Squirrel grinned and patted me on the shoulder.

I rolled my eyes again as I watched Squirrel flip through the local paper. It was an overly humid sunny Saturday, and I did not have to go to the House of Seven Gables to give a tour. My mom would be home in the evening. Squirrel and I had positioned ourselves on the sofa and as close to the blowing air conditioning box wedged in my apartment window as possible.

Squirrel scanned the bottom of the newspaper and flopped down on the sofa.

"Hey Zander, have you seen this advertisement about the local triathlon? You should enter this in a few days. You are perfect for it. You now have the swimming down, you have been biking around all summer, now you just need to do a little jogging. Why not add triathlete to your current résumé of awesomeness? I'm going to coach you to victory, and I will only take ten percent of the $200 top prize for your age group when you win."

"Intense exercise and having diabetes are not a good combination, Squirrel. I could pass out if I run too fast."

"Excuses, excuses. You can't have an excuse mindset. Didn't you do any of that mindfulness at your fancy school? Just set your brain to it and get it done. If you feel week, you can just keep popping candy and sugar tabs as you run. That's why I am the coach, and you will be the trainee," said Squirrel.

Squirrel's eyes bulged. He stood up suddenly.

"I cannot believe you did not tell me it was today!" he almost screamed.

"What?" I said.

"Don't give me that nonsense. You knew today was the first day of filming, and you knew I would forget because I always forget things like this, and it is your job to remind me. You didn't remind me because you don't want to go," Squirrel howled.

"That's exactly right. I don't want to go at all. I don't want to see my father."

"Are you kidding me? This will make us famous. There will be a thousand people there on the set. What are the odds of us bumping into your father? It was meant to be!"

"Too high of a chance for me. He keeps texting me hoping to chat."

"Okay, then do it for me. Do it for your Mom," Squirrel pled.

"Please," I said. "Are you going to list any other family members in this argument?"

"You are guaranteed to get a spot in this film. Look at you. Tall, thin, handsome, local boy. You even know the producer."

"You are nuts, Squirrel. Obviously, you haven't been getting enough attention this summer."

"Let's just go down to the park and see what's going on. What's the harm in that?"

"Are you kidding me? The last time I went to that park, I almost killed a girl on a bike with a flying ice cream freezer. Let's see what could happen...arrest, getting in trouble with my mom, having birds attack me. Should I go on?"

"This is too big of a movie to just sit home. It could be next summer's blockbuster, and you can be a part of it. We should at least go and see what they are filming today. We will be back before lunch."

Squirrel was practically begging me. He pulled my t-shirt until I finally relented.

"Oh, and before we go, please put on your tan tour guide uniform with the cargo shorts from the museum. I think it will help us get into the movie if you are in a full uniform. It will make you stand out. Uniformed people always get on television first."

I rolled my eyes, but I did eventually submit to Squirrel's demands.

He and I parked our bikes at the far end of the Salem Commons Park to not attract any attention. I was fearful that security from the Hawthorne Hotel would recognize me and call the police again. I was doing well as a tour guide but really didn't want to get into any more trouble with the law this summer.

I poked my head around the corner of the brick building to see massive white vans, trailers, and dozens of people moving lights, cables, and cameras around. Squirrel and I made our way over to the park, and I felt a chill as I remembered the last time I was there I drove a truck across the lawn and almost dropped a freezer on a small child.

"No drama," I whispered to myself.

"Did you say something?" Squirrel said.

I shook him off as we crossed the street into the park. There was a large group of teenagers eating cookies and fruit from a long table. I slid in with the teenagers, discreetly gave myself some insulin, and pulled three cookies from the table. I was ridiculously hungry. Squirrel slipped snacks into his backpack by the handful.

"Squirrel, really?"

"Just a few more, these snacks are top quality."

I felt a tapping on my shoulder just as Squirrel was zipping up his backpack. There was an intense sense of dread that ran from the hairs on my arms to my tingling feet. I just promised myself that there would be no more trouble. I just wanted to watch some of the movie. That was it. I slowly turned around toward the tapping.

"Where have you been? I've been calling you."

Movie producer Ernie Reynolds held two phones, a clipboard, and three walkie-talkies were attached to his waist.

"I told you I wanted you in the movie. I have a great part for you. You're a local kid, and it's even better that I saw the article on you in the local paper. That was a big story that should have received more attention."

Squirrel tapped me on the shoulder and nodded.

"See, I told you so. It was a big deal," Squirrel politely reminded me again.

"Well, no time for all this chatter. We have the large chase scene in the park today. There are hundreds of zombies ready to tear the flesh off the locals around here."

Squirrel coughed up some cookie crumbs, and the cookies digesting in my stomach suddenly did not feel so great.

"I love the costume you wore today, Zander. It's very original. It will be perfect," Ernie said.

"Actually, it is authentic." I was pointing to my cargo shorts and museum guide shirt.

"Even better. Let's have you sign this form."

An assistant appeared out of nowhere and handed me a paper to sign.

"You will waive any rights to sue the movie production if you are injured in this zombie attack, but more importantly you will be paid."

Squirrel leaned in behind me. "Remember my ten percent."

"You will receive $200 a day for this extra work, but if the director asks you to say a line of dialogue, even one word, the rate changes."

"Great," I said as I signed the paper.

"It increases to $2,000 per day."

"Ka-ching," said Squirrel. "Keep talking, Zander, and we are in the money!"

The assistant escorted me to a hair and makeup tent.

"What about, my special friend?" I asked the assistant.

"He will be with the rest of the standby extras if we even need them at all. It's up to the director on how many extras he wants to see eaten by zombies today. It will depend on his mood."

Squirrel gave a fist pump to be potentially eaten by zombies. The hairstylist poofed my hair a bit and dabbed some powder on my nose. She said powder made me look better on camera.

I walked over to the center of the park to see a bunch of extras staring at a man holding a microphone.

"I can't believe it's really him," whispered the person next to me.

"Who is he?" I asked.

"He's the director, Henry Whitsmore. Sorry, Sir Henry Whitsmore. He's directed Shakespeare at the Globe Theater and acted in *Hamlet*."

I nodded trying to understand what the extra was saying. "He's a world class director, and now he is here right in front of us!"

"Directing a zombie movie," I said.

"I wouldn't mention that to the director if you want to be paid," said the extra.

Another assistant spritzed my hair and moved from extra to extra while I gazed out at a sea of zombies. Assistant directors were instructing the undead horde how to move slowly, ungracefully but clearly focused on a target. I heard the occasional scream, and two zombies practiced attacking a victim. Somewhere out there in this sea of the undead was my father. This was a man I had not seen in almost three years.

"Talent let's move!" yelled an assistant.

People in the movie biz call actors or even background actors "talent." I guess that's me for the day. We assembled in the middle of the park.

We stood around a well-dressed man wearing a suit and tie. On one side of him was a horde of dripping ravenous zombies dressed in ragged clothes and actors chomping to get into character. I stood on the other side of Sir Whitsmore surrounded by actors dressed as October tourists, kids in Halloween costumes, and fathers holding cameras. Sir Whitsmore held his hands up in the air for attention. The silence was instantaneous.

"Thank you for coming, everyone. Here is the scene for the day. This is the first time our reanimated pioneers of Salem Village have reached the center of the city, here at the Commons. The horde slowly moved from Gallows Hill on the outskirts of the city to where we are now. The horde has been growing hungrier and more ravenous as they march across the unsuspecting town. Too many generations of people have forgotten what happened to its former residents in the 1600s. These zombies now seek revenge for those atrocities. It is the afternoon of

Halloween and unsuspecting parents are out trick or treating with their kids. They do not suspect that some of the costumed locals are actually legitimate zombies."

The director gave the movie's summary with such passion I felt I had to give him my full support even though I had seen about a thousand zombie movies. I knew since I was on the side of the living at the start of this scene my chances were not very good of surviving. It was about a twenty-to-one ratio of zombies to fresh live meat.

"When I call 'action,' the zombies are going to move toward the young couple with the trick or treater. They will have an unpleasant surprise when the zombie chooses the trick over the treat and tears into the dad's arm. The dad will scream, sending loose the army of the undead around him."

The director stopped his speech and locked eyes with me. "Young sir."

I swallowed hard. The director was staring at me.

He walked over to me.

"I love your tour guide outfit. It's splendidly original."

"It is authentic actually," I muttered.

"Brilliant. You will be giving directions to this person."

Sir Whitsmore positioned an extra near me and a prop person handed the other actor a map of the city.

"You can be mouthing directions; remember: no actual talking."

My shoulders slumped. I thought my payday was finally going to arrive. I just needed to say one word in the movie, and I would get $2,000 minus the ten percent I would give Squirrel. The director kept staring at my cargo hat as he positioned all the actors for the scene.

"I'm a bit inspired today. I want you to knock this hat off when you start running away from the zombies. The hat will then fall to the ground."

"Will I get it back? It's property of the museum," I asked.

"I love this boy. You are in the middle of a major motion picture, and you are concerned about your hat. Of course, you will get it back. It might be a little muddy," the director said.

Sir Whitsmore continued. "The hat will fall to the ground, and it will be picked up by one of the undead. The ghoulish soul will examine the hat, and we'll pull in for a close-up to show a glimmer, just a glimmer of recognition. I want to humanize these undead monsters for just a half a second before the total onslaught."

Sir Whitsmore held the hat and surveyed his sea of monsters. He whispered to an assistant who brought over the director's personal step stool. Sir Whitsmore climbed to the top of the step stool and straightened his tie.

"You, my friend with the protruding gash in your head, come forth into the spotlight."

The zombies parted quite peacefully as the chosen one sauntered toward Sir Whitsmore. He gently placed the hat in the zombie's shriveled hands.

"I want you to express just a twinkle of humanity for just a second. The hat has reminded you of your previous life. Give just the twinkle and then return to your ravenous state of being undead."

I had a blocked view as Sir Whitsmore practiced with the zombie.

"That's perfect! This will really add some spice to the start of this scene. Let's get into first position, everyone. I want all three cameras rolling on this one."

The director stepped back to reveal the zombie who would retrieve my hat. I saw a figure with a long gash on his head and disgusting fake teeth. Beneath the layers of makeup, I recognized the face; the eyes were the same as mine. My father had returned.

Zombie Dad turned toward me and was speechless. I wasn't sure if it was because he was wearing false teeth or the fact he had not seen me in years. I was much taller than the little boy he abandoned.

"Zander, I—"

I heard those two words coming out of his mouth. The sentence crawled out from behind yellow, disfigured teeth.

"Quiet everyone, ready for the first take!" Sir Whitsmore yelled from behind a monitor.

I turned away from my father and stood next to the woman holding the map. I pointed to some spots on the map and whispered quiet nonsense words to her. She reciprocated with nonsense words as well. I heard Whitsmore yell "action" and the zombies moved toward the unsuspecting dad with his trick or treating daughter. I kept a corner of my eye on the main action while still directing the lost tourist. The zombie grabbed hold of the father's forearm and took a huge bite.

I was unprepared by how much blood erupted from his arm. The fake blood was flying everywhere, and I felt a splatter across my face. This was gross. Both the little trick or treater and the girl's acting father screamed in unison. This was our cue to turn and run across the field. I turned and brushed my hat off and saw it fall to the ground. I saw Zombie Dad pick it up as the cameras turned toward Dad for his close-up. The screaming little trick or treater who just witnessed her father get chomped ran right into me and knocked me down into the mud. I got up quickly to feel a sharp pain in my ankle. I thought I'd twisted it. Searing pain had already reached my brain. I was covered in mud and fake blood. Zombie Dad lurched toward me, holding my blood-soaked hat. I climbed away from him, but a meandering zombie could outrun a twisted ankle, blood splattered middle-schooler any day.

I didn't hear Sir Whitsmore call a "cut" on the scene as Dad was right on top of me. The scene was still being filmed. Zombie Dad reached out and handed me the hat. His disfigured face leered over me, and I erupted.

"I don't want the stupid hat back!" I gave him a hard push, and I tried to limp away from him. He let out an incoherent moaning sound. Dad was a bit stunned and strolled forward not slowing down. I became even angrier and kicked him in the shin.

Zombie Dad showed his decomposed teeth while letting out a huge hiss, trying to stifle his human yell.

"Stupid jerk!" I turned and hobbled away to try to catch up with the other screaming humans.

"Cut!" yelled Sir Whitsmore.

The zombies stopped moaning.

"That was great, guys. Have that kid come back here. We may use that take and his line or maybe change the line on the second take. I need a contract for him right now."

Sir Whitsmore snapped his fingers for an assistant to go fetch me.

I kept limping off the field toward the snack table. I could hear the director yelling for me to return. I saw Squirrel. His shorts were loaded with snacks, and his cheeks were puffed out with food. He was hopping up and down yelling.

"Payday, payday, good buddy."

I limped all the way out of the park.

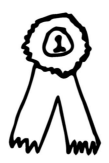

CHAPTER TWELVE
Everyone's a Winner

Squirrel was sitting in his usual spot on my sofa counting a pile of twenty-dollar bills. He spread the wad of money across his hand and started fanning himself.

"This feels so good. Two thousand dollars for yelling at your Dad. I still can't believe it. You got paid to yell at your deadbeat Zombie Dad. I get two hundred dollars for just dragging your sad self to the park. This was my most profitable gig ever. We went from collecting cans on the beach to sitting on easy money!"

Squirrel flopped back on the sofa and counted his money again.

I shook my head and just mindlessly played on my phone.

"What genius it was to trip, fall into the mud, and start howling at Mr. Burke, and then the director went crazy about what he saw. He loved it. He said to the crew it added authenticity to the scene. Who worries about being authentic in a zombie chase scene? Unbelievable."

Squirrel continued to fan himself with his spread-out money. His smile was almost contagious.

He tapped his phone. "This is our training day today, Zander. You said you would try the triathlon tomorrow, and I would get a ten-percent cut again. It won't be nearly as much of a payday as the movie, but money is money. We have a few more days off until the movie production needs you again."

I stood up out of my chair and stretched. My ankle felt much better. Mom had been telling me to get more exercise, especially since I had to play an afternoon sport for grade six. It was a physical education requirement that I play some sports for the entire school year. My September choices were soccer and cross-country, and I was not good at either one. The last time I played an organized sport was when I hit a baseball off a rubber tee and ran to first base. When I reached first base I could jump up and down on it. The base made a loud squeaking noise. It had helped young players remember where to run and infuriated fans listening to loud squeaking the entire game.

"Here's the deal, Zander. You are going to swim one length of Dead Horse Beach. You remember that was the beach where the hawk attacked you."

"Seagull. I remember very clearly."

"Maybe you can ride that ghost horse Wildfire across the water to the finish line," said Squirrel.

"I may need a horse to finish this race," I said.

"Seriously, here is the route. After you swim the length of the beach, you are going to bike four miles. Go past the cat lady's house where you had your daring rescue," Squirrel said.

"Okay. I know that area too."

"Finally, you are going to run two miles around the park and the arcade. It's going to be easy squeezy. There is a $200-dollar prize for twelve and unders. You will be running against little squirts since you are the oldest looking kid in the city."

"I've never been big into doing strenuous activity for a few hours, Squirrel. It's tough to manage the diabetes."

"Are you kidding me? You are going to play the lame diabetes card on me? You said you would never use that excuse with me. I am going to disqualify that response, big goofball. You told me to smack you in the head if you ever used diabetes as a reason to get out of anything. I'm going to smack you in the head right now. Be ready."

Squirrel came right up to me.

I put up my fists in self-defense as Squirrel threw a few air jabs but did not come close to my head.

"I really said that?"

Squirrel nodded his head affirmatively. "Many times."

"It's just tough to manage low blood sugar under all that continuous exercise. You know it sends my blood sugar number into a downward spiral when I am constantly moving. Mix in the stress of the race and the heat, and you may find me passed out on the floor again."

I have always said that diabetes is a part of me. The disease does not define me, nor does it limit me. I would not let this happen. I guess I was out of excuses with my agent, Mr. Squirrel.

"Okay, I am ready," I said. I needed a distraction away from my constantly texting Zombie Dad in town, and the fact I still did not want to respond to any of his messages. He was trying to bribe me with a trip to a fancy restaurant, Legos, comics, or a go-cart racing trip. I still did not want to talk to him.

"Great. Let's do a little training. My surefire, get-fit-quick regimen you are going to follow starts in just a few minutes. First, you are going to run on the sidewalk, and I am going to chase you on my bike. If my bike tire hits your foot, this means you need to run faster. It's very simple, run…"

"Or be run over," I continued. "What kind of motivational coach are you? Trying to maul your one and only client?"

"I'm motivated by money, dinero. Haven't you figured that out yet?"

Squirrel stood up and folded his money in his pocket. He picked a crumb of food off his shirt, sniffed it for a second, and then put it in his mouth. "And motivated by food."

I had an afternoon of relentless training with Squirrel. I ran; he chased me and tried to rub his tire into my heels as often as he could. I swam, and he paddled after me in an inner tube and hit my face with a squirt gun. I will give Squirrel credit. He will do anything for a payday, and he was making me push myself faster and harder and not forgetting to give me some sugar pills or a large gulp of an energy drink.

The next morning, I was standing in the ice-cold ocean with water up to my knees. The small chalkboard on the lifeguard's chair read a frosty water temperature of only fifty-eight degrees. It was like stepping into a shower the minute you turn it on. I thought my body would adjust to the temperature, but my feet felt a little numb.

I couldn't believe I was doing this. Squirrel gave me a big wave from the beach while I continued to shiver and was surrounded by boys and girls much smaller than me. I felt like a big tuna in a sardine can until I felt a tap on my shoulder.

"Zander, it's great to see you. I can't believe you're here."

I turned behind me to see my fifth-grade classmate, Brady Wiggins. Brady radiated vitality like he had just stepped out of a sports catalog. His hair was perfect, and he was wearing a tight body suit. I had not seen him since he carried my semiconscious body into murse Liam's room.

I felt the loose fabric of my not so fashionable bacon strip designed bathing suit. "What's with the body suit, Brady?"

"You like this? My mom just bought it for me. It's supposed to be aerodynamic and help me with biking and running. It is made from moisture wicking fabric, so it will be practically dry the second I come out of the water. I won't even need a towel to dry off before I get on my bike. The water just magically leaves my body."

"You mean evaporates?" I said.

"Sure, whatever you said," Brady responded.

I gave a squeeze of my shirt to get some of the water out of it. My shirt already felt like it weighed fifty pounds.

"Man, Zander, I am going to beat this record for the twelve and unders. That prize money is going to come in handy. What are you going to use the prize money for, Zander?

"Groceries."

"Ah, Zander, always a kidder." Brady slapped me on the back. I wasn't kidding.

"I think I'm going to upgrade the data plan on my device to get high definition streaming anytime, anywhere, or buy some vintage sneakers. It's really too difficult to decide," Brady lamented.

"I can't decide between bread and milk or just milk. Decisions, decisions." I was being a bit snarky and didn't really care. I had it up to about my freezing bacon shorts with Brady's condescending remarks. It was bad enough to endure his comments all school year but hearing them in the middle of the summer was practically inhumane.

"Swimmers take your position!" yelled the announcer over a bullhorn. "You are to swim the length of the beach and come out at the far end and head to your bike for the second leg of the race. If you can't swim, you need to stay behind the swimmers or walk in at least waist-deep water to keep it fair and equitable."

"What kind of twelve-year-old doesn't know how to swim? He or she shouldn't even be in this competition!" Brady said.

"It's just for fun, isn't it?" I asked.

"You keep telling yourself that, Zander, as I blow past you. See you at the finish line. I will be drinking my protein shake. It helps me recover faster."

I wanted to dump a protein shake on his enlarged head.

I heard a siren go off, and the shoving from behind started immediately. I belly flopped into the water and started a freestyle swimming move. Brady moved like a fish in its natural habitat and expertly maneuvered around the other kids and slithered away. I felt a couple of close brushes of feet against my face and saw kids running along the shoreline. They were not walking in waist-level water.

I kept my head above water as I transitioned from a freestyle swim to a doggie paddle. It wasn't pretty, but I just wanted to get out of the water without getting kicked in the teeth. I reached the end of the beach, and there was a path cleared on the sand that led to the bike area. I came out of the water with sand wedging between my toes. I could see Brady reaching the bike pit. The crowd was cheering me on, and I saw Squirrel waving me to the bike pit. I felt the first wave of low blood sugar start to hit me. I felt a little dizzy but not enough to stop. I didn't see a snack stop anywhere and didn't want to slow down.

I reached the roped off bike area. Parents were discouraged from helping their children get on their bikes or wipe off sand. Brady's bike was next to mine. His bike was another item practically out of a professional racing shop. It was black, spotless, and had more gears and attachments on it than I'd ever thought possible. Mine was the one found under an overpass or tossed out of a van by the side of the road. Mom never got around to the bike upgrade I had been hoping for. I had the seat up as far as I could without it popping out of the frame. The bike used to be gray, but it had large chunks of rust confusing the overall color. It was a bike that didn't need a high-tech braking system. It had one, my feet. It was those same feet that pushed the pedals backward to make the bike stop. My kneecaps shifted slightly outward instead of forward to move the bike. I figured that the bike had one last good race in it before it was recycled into a toaster.

Brady was already on his bike and peddling away by the time I reached my old clunker. Brady was perfectly dry while I was still soaking wet. I saw his perfectly molded individual toe sneakers peddle off down the street.

Having diabetes can be problematic during extreme exercise. I don't have the ability to add any stored sugar from my liver and muscles into my bloodstream. To put it simply, I need sugar fast when I am exercising heavily. I bet I was at a blood glucose number quickly dropping to 50 when my goal was 125 by the time I sat on my bike. I was just guessing since I was getting pretty good at how my body was feeling. I didn't have my kit on me, so I didn't have a way to check my exact number. The slight dizziness told me I was low and fading fast. I peddled up the first hill of the four-mile bike race. I was speeding past my competition with my legs moving quickly but still a little out, so I wouldn't bump into my handlebars. I made it down the hill and finally saw the water station. I was hoping they had more than water since water would cool me down but not help a crashing blood sugar. I really didn't need another trip to the hospital this summer.

I hit the foot brake hard and skidded to a stop right in front of the water stand. I scanned the small cups of water. Searching, searching. I spotted a few cups of Gatorade at the end of the table. I grabbed one in each hand.

"Just try to take one, honey," said the attendant.

"I have diabetes."

She didn't say anything. I didn't expect her to. Most people don't know what to say or have very little knowledge about the disease when I say the disease's name aloud. I realized a long time ago that I had to rely primarily on myself. I didn't realize until this summer that I was terrible in my routine and needed to make changes to be healthier. I didn't want to be one of those people with diabetes and a missing toe.

The attendant just nodded as I sucked down the sugary sweetness. I tossed the cups on the ground and peddled away to finish the first mile. The drink was like an instant bolt of life. I went from lethargic and dizzy to ready to conquer the world. My groggy body caught up with my mind. The sugar kicking in is like when you find one of those cool dimmer lights in a pitch-black room. You slowly move it from pitch black gently up to reveal a bright luminescence.

I made it back to the bike pit after four miles and felt like I might need some more sugar. I had been pushing it hard on my bike for a while. I parked my bike and saw Brady squeezing his stomach. I couldn't believe I caught up to him.

"Man, Zander. You are fast today. I have a killer cramp."

"Sorry to hear that, Brady." I started running out of the pit for the final two miles of the triathlon. Brady caught up to me.

"I had a huge carbohydrate load before the race. Pasta, bagels, you name it. I scarfed it down. I can't shake this cramp right now. What did you eat?"

"Some juice and yogurt, not much in the fridge," I responded.

"Smart man as always, Zander. See you at the finish line." Brady bolted away from me still clutching his side.

By the second mile I felt I had consumed my weight in Gatorade. It was a full-blown balancing act to maintain the extreme exercise while keeping my blood sugar up. I felt like I was in a good spot since I seemed to be passing quite a few kids and only a few were passing me. I finally caught up to Brady who was still squeezing his stomach. He was slowing down as my feet were hitting the pavement hard in the final mile.

We were side by side with the finish line in sight when a small boy who was ahead of us tripped and fell onto the asphalt road. Brady shrugged upon seeing the boy with seriously bruised knees and scraped hands.

"Just leave him, Zander. It's you and me in a one-on-one footrace to the finish line."

I saw the kid ahead of us trying to get up. We were almost on top of him. It didn't feel right to me as I saw Brady swerve around this human traffic accident. I came to a sudden stop, and my legs screamed for halting so suddenly. I saw Brady shake his head at me and continued toward the finish line. I helped the small boy up.

"Are you okay? What's your name?" I asked.

"Billy."

Figures. What a coincidence. A genuine Billy only after I said goodbye to my fictional one. I helped Billy up, and he limped as we did a fast walk toward the finish. Billy was really leaning on me as we crossed the finish line. Billy's mother thanked me profusely as she shuffled him off to the nurse's station. A finish line attendant put a medal around my neck as I moved to the snack area. I could see Squirrel helping himself to some of the post-race bananas, protein drinks, and granola bars.

Brady walked up to me flashing his medal.

"Finished on top, Zander!" He peered at my medal.

"Ha, participant! They give those medals to any chump in the race.

You could finish last and still get that same medal. You blew your chances for a finalist medal and some prize money by helping that kid. How does that make you feel?"

I looked past Brady's gleaming first place medal to see Billy at the nurse's station.

"I'm really fine with it, Brady. I gave it my best."

"Really, your best?"

Brady didn't understand the internal struggle I had against my own body this afternoon. It wasn't his problem. It was mine. Maybe it was finally time to get an insulin pump.

"It really was my best, Brady."

I turned to walk away. Then, I stopped and said, "I'll see you in sixth grade, Brady."

I headed to the snack table to try to stop Squirrel from stuffing more snacks into his shorts. He brought his extra-long shorts with the deep pockets just for this situation.

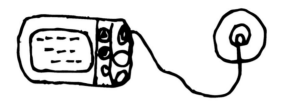

CHAPTER THIRTEEN
Talk to your Doctor

"Zander are you ready to wear an insulin pump?"

I nodded yes. I sat in the small room at Salem Hospital and answered Dr. Berard's questions. He was teaching a class my mom was taking and was the head of the endocrinology department. Endocrinology is the study of a person's glands and hormones. Diabetes falls into this category, so this is the wing of the hospital that I visited too often. I felt like I was getting a bit of special attention with Dr. Berard walking me through the setup of the small device, how to fill it, and how to attach it to my stomach. I wasn't ready to wear a glucose monitoring device but did want something that would give me a break from all the needles. Mom had pulled a few strings to get me the latest pump technology.

Dr. Berard watched as I clipped the phone sized item onto my shorts and put the clear tube against my stomach. He helped as I connected the end of the tube to an infusion site on my stomach. The infusion site had a small needle that politely dug into my belly. Once the tube was connected to this site, I could then tell the pump to send insulin through the tube and directly into my body. My years of constant needle injections were almost over. This device would give me a more consistent flow of insulin and hopefully not have so many high blood sugar numbers.

The triathlon was the final blow to me agreeing to an insulin pump permanently. I was tired of the constant highs and lows and thought this new device would keep me at an even level. I had fought for so long to not have a pump, but I needed to have more control in my already downward spiraling life.

I will have to change the entry spot on my stomach every three days. If I wanted to get a donut with Squirrel I just pressed a button on the pump, and it was instant medicine. The device was about the size of an old flip phone and delivered the medicine instantaneously. Easy peazy.

"Thanks for doing this, Dr. Berard. I appreciate you doing this for me and my mom."

Dr. Berard smiled and took his time reviewing my chart. "We ran your A1C level from the blood sample we took when you came in today, and it is slightly better than it was back in the spring."

My A1C measured how much concentrated glucose or sugar was attached to the hemoglobin in the red blood cells in my bloodstream. It was very dangerous to have high levels of glucose in my or anyone's blood. By giving myself more insulin, it reduced the sugar buildup in my blood. High blood sugar would lead to future health issues that I just didn't want.

"Keep doing what you are doing, Zander. Your numbers are slightly better. I know your mom is relieved you are now on the pump, but, most importantly, are you feeling well about this?"

Is a middle schooler ever satisfied with anything for long? It could be Bigfoot dancing with unicorns one minute to everyone hates me the next. I was dealing with my health issues, and my Zombie Dad was still terrorizing the town and couldn't stop trying to reach me. I made some money this summer but not as much as I had hoped. I felt like I'd failed more than I'd succeeded.

"I'm satisfied with it, Dr. Berard. I like the device, and I am ready to try my best."

"I'm glad to hear this, Zander. I won't see you for another two weeks. If you are ready to get on with your day, can you help me in a little matter in the hospital?"

I nodded affirmatively. Dr. Berard escorted me out of the patient room and down to the intensive care unit. I was hoping I could be a doctor for the day like some of my classmates were able to be principal for the day. Maybe he heard about how I was helping my mom out with the money or my speaking part in the movie.

Dr. Berard pulled back the curtain to reveal a small boy in bed with an IV drip hooked up to his arm. His mother sat in a chair next to his bed. The boy turned to me, and his eyes lit up. His mother gave a smile.

"It's you!" said the boy.

I didn't think I would ever see him again.

Dr. Berard reviewed his chart. "This is Billy and his mother, Mrs. Andrews. Billy came in yesterday and was diagnosed with type 1 diabetes. I like to have some of our more experienced experts with diabetes talk to the young patients for a few minutes. It looks like you might even know Billy."

"I do. We met once before," I said.

Billy sat up in bed. "He helped me at the end of the race when I took a fall. I was going to be trampled by all these kids."

Billy's mom smiled.

"Zander was quite heroic, and Billy could not stop talking about him and now, well, here you are!" said Mrs. Andrews. "What a ridiculously small world."

"I thought Zander could share some good information with you, Billy. Zander has been a patient here for almost three years and is now on an insulin pump. He's getting to be a top-notch patient with his personal care and health. He is really figuring out the nuances of this disease."

I lifted my shirt just a little bit to show the clear tube across my stomach and ending at a band aid near my belly button. Dr. Berard left the room and closed the door. Mrs. Andrews and Billy focused their full attention on me. I started to get nervous. I tapped my foot a few times.

"So, Billy, how have you been after the race?"

"That was just one of the many dizzy spells I'd been having. I thought I was just hot and having to go to the bathroom all the time, so we finally went to the hospital. The doctors and nurses told me it wasn't an accident that I fell at the end of the race. I got dizzy. The doctor said I was having 'fatigue.'"

"Yeah, when I was first diagnosed as having diabetes I was fatigued, sleepy, and had some blurred vision. By the time I left the hospital I was in good shape."

I thought about all the times I had experienced lows this summer and had been unprepared for them. I put myself in too many dangerous situations. I didn't want to get Billy too scared about what could happen in his future.

"Billy, it's your job to keep your numbers in the low 100s through good checking, exercise, and healthy eating choices."

I sounded like a commercial, but I had been making some poor choices over the past few years and didn't want Billy to plummet down the same chasm.

Mrs. Andrews was flipping through all the diabetes pamphlets given to her.

"Zander, do you have many lows?"

I thought about stumbling outside the comic book store and the fall in the Chinese house. Those were just the recent ones.

"I still do have some lows. It's part of life. Just make sure you have a strategy. Strategy is key."

Billy nodded to everything I was saying.

"I was diagnosed almost three years ago, and it gets better every year. In my case, the disease can become predictable. I'm ready to take on sixth grade at Flowing Meadows."

"Flowing Meadows? That's where Billy is going for first grade," said his mother.

"Excellent. I will be in another building but will come over to check on you. We insulin craving creatures need to stick together."

I reached out and fist pumped Billy.

"The hospital is going to give you a mountain of supplies. It will be hard at first but before you know it, you will be a major movie star like me," I said.

"Are you in the zombie movie, Zander?" Billy asked.

"I have a small role but have to go back tomorrow for the final zombie attack scene."

"Cool," said Billy.

"What's even cooler is all this technology," I said.

I pulled my shirt up again to show him my small insulin pump. I pointed to the tube running from the device to my stomach. Billy reached up out of bed and lightly touched the clear tube.

"This pump is state of the art." I showed Billy the app on my phone. "I can punch in whatever I need right from my phone. I don't need to give myself shots anymore. I bet you have had quite a few of those needles the past few days while in the hospital."

Billy showed me a light bruise on his arm.

"Every time I eat or even have a snack," Billy said. He flopped back down in exasperation against his pillow.

"You might eventually get one of these once you figure out what your body needs. Remember, you can do anything you want. Let yourself eat that piece of birthday cake covered in frosting at the party. Don't let people say you can't have a type of food because you have diabetes. If you take the right amount of insulin, you can have the food. It's very simple. Just remember that, little man."

"I will, Zander."

Mrs. Andrews stood up and gave me a huge hug. I was more of a handshake guy with adults, but I allowed it in this case. She made me sit down on Billy's bed as she snapped a picture of the two of us.

"This was a big help, Zander. You are a great role model."

I never pictured myself as a role model to anyone. I felt like a complete failure this summer, but visiting Billy gave me a little hope. My imaginary brother, Billy, had only recently left to now return as a real Billy and someone I really could help. The film shoot was tomorrow, and I was going to confront Zombie Dad.

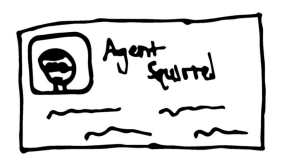

CHAPTER FOURTEEN
The Witches Apocalypse

No Squirrel, no Mom, no backup, no distractions. It was just me against an army of zombies ready to rip apart my hometown. The zombified victims from the Salem Witch Trials of 1693 had returned to Salem seeking revenge on the present-day population. I was going to be with the film's main character by the name of Owen and his perfectly combed hair. The zombies were particularly annoyed with Owen and wished to tear him apart chunk by chunk. Sir Whitsmore's assistant sent me an email yesterday and allowed me to read the entire script to help me get into character. My character, "Slim," had a main goal not to be eaten and to run in the opposite direction of the zombies as fast as possible.

The email showed up on my phone last night while Mom was helping me change my pump site. It was the third day with my tube on a specific spot on my stomach, so I had to refill the small device with insulin and pick a new spot on my stomach to stick the needle and secure the tape. I was extremely systematic about changing my sites and didn't want any bruising or infection. Once I was done, I felt a bit relieved. I was good to go for the next three days. This would get me through the ending of the film shoot and an encounter with my father. My phone gave a loud buzz, and I read the message marked "urgent" sent from the film director's assistant. It was the entire movie script. I had been piecing the story together since I'd met the producer Ernie in the hotel last month and my first scene at the park. Squirrel had been trolling web sites to get the plot, but I didn't want to read anything unofficial.

The entire script was sent on an app that would erase the file the minute I read the last page. The production company was vigilant about keeping the movie's plot a surprise until people paid to watch it next summer.

I sat on my bed with some pretzels, half a bar of chocolate, and I read the entire script. It took me almost two hours to read it, and the script erased itself as promised after I scrolled over the words "The End" on the last page. I was surprised that it was actually a pretty good story. I thought it might be like some zombie-of-the-week or shark-attack made-for-TV movie, but I would consider paying some of my hard-earned cash to see it in an adjustable chair and air-conditioned theater next summer. I might be able to save my ticket money and be invited to the red-carpet premiere at the local theater since a movie theater was one of the few places where I did not run into trouble this summer. I felt like I had to get into the mindset of the helpless victim, Slim, and be ready to give it my all. I was told by the production to be prepared to do some screaming and maybe a few more words in the final attack. The sound of a cash register went off in my head minus the ten percent for my agent, Mr. Squirrel.

I laughed when I saw Squirrel's handmade business cards stating "Agent" on it and his ten percent commission. He specialized in getting "ginormous bucks from gigantic projects" and a "payday now" with only a rudimentary drawing of a squirrel holding a cellphone. Squirrel's direct number was listed below the drawing. He was actively attempting to get more clients in the area.

Mom made sure I had my House of Seven Gables outfit pressed and ready. She had even brought it to the dry cleaners. Mom worked out the details with the museum to make sure I could wear the uniform in the movie. I was told logos and official companies had to be "pre-approved," and Mom said it was all set with my boss. My boss at the museum said she would even count my hours at the film shoot as community service hours since I was advertising the museum by wearing the uniform. It was a double bonus for me to get paid and get my service hours done, if I didn't get in trouble with the police again.

I took my bike down to the Salem Willows Amusement Park. The park had a row of arcade shops, kiddie rides, pizza, Chinese, and seafood establishments. The sidewalk in front of the amusement park was roped off with caution tape separating actors from many local onlookers hoping to see the imminent zombie attack.

I parked and locked my bike to a stop sign pole and made my way to the check-in area for actors. I could smell the breakfast food drifting toward me. I checked in by giving my name, "Zander Burke." I was told to be ready for the director's speech in about an hour and have breakfast quickly. Hair and makeup personnel would come by and check on me. I made the turn toward the food table.

"Hey, how come you get food?"

I turned to see a helmet camera shining right in my face.

"You again. The kid who broke my VR gloves."

Bruce, the heavyset technology expert, moved his helmet cam closer to my face.

"Thanks, kid. The insurance from when you pushed me down that hidden staircase allowed me to upgrade my VR gear. Do you know how much publicity I gained from that old house incident? I am all plugged in once again and have been documenting the behind the scenes on this zombie film shoot in Salem all summer. You are in a bit too much of my documentary. I saw you pitch a fit in the mud and limp away from that zombie. The zoom-in on this helmet camera is amazing. I have quite a bit of footage on you, Zander. It's highly enlightening."

"What do you mean?"

"You'll see. You seem to generate positive responses from my fan base. I have no idea why. I would label you as a straight up juvenile delinquent, but thousands of my followers make comments about you managing your diabetes and being a good kid. Only time and the internet will tell who is right, Zander."

He knew very little about me, yet he was blabbing his opinions about me to all his followers. I was being judged by the unknown. Bruce blew a breath over his virtual reality gloves, giving them a perfect gleaming shine.

"I will have a screening of my behind the scenes documentary at the Salem Theater next summer, or maybe I will stream it online for a small fee. It will be a great fan point of view on this Hollywood blockbuster or complete failure of a movie."

Bruce waved all his gear toward me and filmed the entire actor's area. "I told you I was sorry about the accident at the museum, and it wasn't a push. I was trying to help you. You were falling backward, and I didn't want you to get hurt. I'm sorry you are so mad at me, but you have to move on."

"You don't have the right to tell me to 'move on.' I just got that ridiculous speech taped. I am going to make a musical mash-up of all the outrageous things you have said to me and post it. I will send you the link. You are priceless, Zander, priceless."

I turned away and headed toward the breakfast table. I finished my breakfast of bacon with a side of even more bacon before being called over to the middle of the arcade room. A small number of well-groomed actors waited until the director, Sir Henry Whitsmore, came into the room. He reviewed the script for the day and passed it to his assistant.

"Welcome, everyone. Thank you for being here this morning. I really value our supporting cast in this film. You have all added a great amount of authenticity to this movie, and I thank you from the bottom of my heart. Many of you will meet our film's star, Jonathan Bishop, otherwise known as the lead character, Owen. He will come into the arcade as part of a scene prior to the last stand on the pier down the road. Owen is trying to lead the zombies to the water where he has a friend who will detonate the pier."

Did he just say detonate the pier? I remembered reading the script; I just assumed the explosion would be done on computer. Not the real thing. The director stayed silent while the cast took in this information.

"So, you all know the end of the movie, and I trust you will keep it a secret until next summer when you pay for a ticket and take everyone, and I mean everyone, you know to see it."

There was a laugh in the arcade room.

"Okay, Owen will come in trying to hide from the zombies as they make their way down the sidewalk toward the pier. This plan will fail because the zombies fully take over this arcade. A few of you will get earplugs because some of these arcade machines are fakes and will explode during the scene. It will add more authenticity if you don't know which machines will explode. I really want to see a truly terrified reaction. It shows much better on film."

Exploding arcade machines? I was hoping that this would go well. I reached down into my pocket to silence my phone. I saw that I had three messages just this morning from Zombie Dad.

Zombie Dad was just going to have to wait for me until after the shoot like I hadn't waited long enough to see him. I stood next to Owen while the director and crew stood behind the camera. I checked my pump to make sure all was well before the big scene. A prop person adjusted my hat to make sure it would not fall off my head during all the action. A stunt man came over and handed me some small earplugs.

"Put these in. You are going to need them," he whispered.

"Really?"

"Really. You don't want your ears to bleed later, do you?"

I put the small earplugs in, and they were totally invisible. I needed to stand behind Owen and expect the unexpected. I felt a brushing against my wide hat and turned toward the tickle. The man-bun dad turned toward me. It was him again from the ice cream store. He was one of the zombie survivors.

"You never showed up!" he yelled.

"What?" My earplugs made it sound like I was listening underwater.

"Can you repeat that?"

"You disrespected me in front of my son!"

"I'm sorry, I didn't want to lose my job!" I responded.

"Well, I respect that, but I still feel like punching you."

"YOU NEED TO WORK ON YOUR RAGE ISSUES. BUT RIGHT NOW, WE SHOULD BE REACTING TO ZOMBIES." Man-bun dad nodded and returned to his spot for filming.

Sir Henry Whitsmore yelled for the actors and crew to be ready.

"Action!"

"Come on everyone, follow me!" yelled Owen.

I stood behind Owen as he herded me and a few other survivors toward the center of the arcade. Suddenly there was a large groan. It came from behind a row of pinball machines. The wall exploded in a cloud of dust. I covered my eyes with my hands to see a hoard of zombies rush in toward us, and some pinball machines were laying on their sides. One zombie pushed a machine over, and it crashed violently against man-bun dad. A hoard of zombies smothered him.

Another pinball machine fell down into pieces right at my feet. I moved past a broken pile of bulbs and wires and tapped it with my foot. It was light as a feather. The machines in the room were props. The pinball machines were all lit up well but could have been flung right at me and not caused any broken bones.

The zombies continued to flounder into the room, and I stayed behind Owen. He grabbed the leg of one of the pinball machines and swung it across a zombie's face. From my angle, I could see that he missed, but with some movie magic the zombie took a hard fall onto some soft cushions away from the view of the cameras. A second zombie trudged even closer to us. Owen reached down to the floor and grabbed an electrical cord with sparks coming out of it.

Owen gripped the sparkling cord and rammed it into the neck of the oncoming zombie. Sparks flew everywhere as the zombie's body twisted and convulsed. It fell to the floor.

"Quick, while we have a chance!" yelled Owen.

He shuffled us out the back of the arcade toward the water and the awaiting pier. I could see that the second wave of zombies was being led by Zombie Dad.

"Cut!" yelled Sir Whitsmore.

Owen stopped running, and a phalanx of assistants dabbed his head, handed him water, and brushed his clothes. He was immediately given a towel and some cold water. I didn't have anyone rushing over to me. I wiped the smoke out of my eyes and felt sweat forming under my armpits. I should stop using cheap deodorant. I walked back to the start of the scene and saw the punched zombie get up off the floor mat and brush himself off. The second one pulled the cord out of the side of his neck and handed it back to the prop person.

"That was wonderful. We are going to do that again. We need an hour to reset the room with the wall and the machines. On this second take, I want you, Mr. Museum Guide Boy with the nice cargo hat."

Sir Whitsmore was pointing to me. I pointed at myself to make sure he really wanted me out of a room full of people.

"Yes, young man, one of our few local survivors. I want you to scream as the wall comes down, and the pinball machine crashes near you. You had quite a horrified, realistic expression."

I didn't want to tell the director that I wasn't acting. I was quite horrified and was prepared to be crushed by an arcade machine in a room filled with zombies.

"I want to see that reaction one more time and let out a scream. Camera Two frame up his reaction shot, we may use it in post-production."

A camera operator came over to start measuring the distance from the camera to my face. I was wondering if a scream counted as a line of dialogue in a movie. I was hoping to get one more $2,000 payday before this movie ended.

The second take and my close-up scream went well, and then we had to break for lunch. I could not believe how slowly shooting a film went. The whole crew relocated to a wooden pier that extended over the ocean. I leaned over the wooden railing and squinted to see the house of my therapist. Her cat, Mr. Cuddles, was probably lurking around the lawn somewhere causing trouble.

The Salem pier was located just beyond the arcade and a row of restaurants. The often-visited landmark stretched over 300 feet or more than a football field over turbulent waves and frigid water. This wooden pier was held up by hundreds of supporting columns descending deep into the earth. I could not believe that it was going to be blown up in the film's finale. I had my trusty cargo hat on and was being sprinkled with spots of blood by a makeup person. Since I was attacked in the last scene, I had to be covered in some tasteful splotches of blood for this upcoming scene. We were picking up with a scene a few minutes after the arcade. I wasn't involved in the last scene. I was told that so much of the movie was filmed out of order and then put together during editing.

I did know that this was going to be my last filmed scene for the character, Slim. During lunch, a production assistant informed me I would be receiving a partial actor rate for my screaming in the arcade.

"A partial rate?" I asked, as I stuffed my face with a roast beef sandwich.

"Yes, 50% pay. It will only be $1,000."

I almost choked on my sandwich. A thousand dollars for yelling? I wish I could do this all the time. If my mom paid me for all the yelling I have done in my lifetime I would be a millionaire.

I nodded politely to the production assistant as she verified my mailing address and moved on to talk to the other actors.

Three thousand dollars earned for just a few days of filming. This movie was my saving grace this summer. I still had to give Squirrel his agent fee of ten percent. I didn't feel badly about giving Squirrel that much money even when I was doing all the work, and he was constantly sneaking around the actor's food table eating and stuffing treats into his pockets. This movie was satisfying his two fundamental needs in life: money and snacks. He was the only friend that gave me a kick in the pants to come to the filming and get off my sorry sofa.

I didn't know how I was going to be safe on the pier with a giant explosion coming up. The prop person came over again and handed me my earplugs. I stood behind Owen when the director yelled action. Owen started walking backward and shuffled me behind him as we headed toward the end of the pier. The sound of the waves crashing against those wooden posts was getting louder and louder as we kept walking backward toward the wooden railing ending the pier. A crowd of about twenty zombies moaned and flailed their outstretched arms. Their slackened jaws and dripping skin were getting closer and closer. Owen reached into his pocket and pulled out a device with a button on it.

"Return to where you came from. We will honor your sacrifice and not forget you!"

A lead character holding a small red device with a button on it usually meant one thing. I had seen enough movies and TV shows to know to be far away from a device like that. My problem was I was standing right next to Owen while he held the device high in the air. I heard the crashing waves below me. I could jump, but it was a very far drop. It might be a death drop. I didn't want to chance it.

Owen put his thumb on a red button, and I guessed that would be it. What a short, miserable life. Too much unsaid, too much time online, and too much self-loathing. If I made it out of this, I was going to be more positive and take better control of my life and my disease.

Owen continued to hold the detonator high in the air while the zombies just stared at him. How could I get off this pier and save my life? I put both hands over my mouth and started screaming. Owen's thumb pressed down on the detonator just as I saw the second row of zombies stop moving and only the first row stepped forward. As soon as the first row stepped onto a dark plank of wood, it crumpled just like the Styrofoam arcade machines.

Fireworks shot out from beneath the pier creating explosions all around me. It was like the Fourth of July with the pops and snaps and all the smoke too. The five zombies in the first row fell through the floor onto a giant inflatable cushion floating on the water under the pier. I thought the whole pier was being blown up when it was just a few fake wooden floorboards. Once again Director Whitsmore received a full-blown realistic performance from me because I really thought the whole pier was going to explode with me standing on it.

"Everyone stays in character, continue the action!" yelled Sir Henry. "We are still rolling cameras."

A few zombies flopped over the open ground to allow a bridge of the undead to be formed. The second wave was pushing us against the back of the pier with multiple cameras filming the fighting between humans and zombies. Owen stepped off to the side to leave me unprotected, and the only zombie I really feared was right in front of me. Zombie Dad.

Zombie Dad tilted his head like I had seen him do it on TV, and his action figure could do this too. It must have been what landed him the part because he owned this character. I could tell it was my father staring at me because of his light blue eyes. He dressed like the undead, but his eyes had not changed. I was pressed against the railing of the pier with nothing but a potential death drop into the crashing waves.

Zombie Dad slowly reached both hands out toward me like he was going to give me a long overdue hug. Did Dad really want to give me that much needed affection during a zombie affliction? With the cameras rolling and an excessive number of people watching us, I thought this would be a slightly unusual time for a father-son reunion. His arms kept rising and stopped by my neck. This was going to be awkward. He put both his hands on my neck. Definitely awkward. Dad squeezed my neck. I started screaming. He was choking me. In front of all these people, my own father was choking the life force out of me. He was the one that ran out on me and my mom, and this was how it all ended? Suffocated by my own Zombie Dad at the end of a pier? He was forcefully moving my neck side to side, and things were getting blurry. I let out a tooth chattering scream again until I heard Sir Henry yell cut.

"That was perfect!" he came out from behind a camera and clapped his hands together. "Very well done. A genuine performance."

Zombie Dad gently pulled his hands away from my neck. I was just as tall as him. He picked up my hat and placed it delicately on my head.

"We need to talk," Dad said.

"I know."

The final take went well with Dad getting smashed in the head by a survivor. I was one of the few survivors still standing in the last scene and anxious to see the final version of the film next summer. Technically, I could still be alive for a sequel. I shook the director's hand and was able to get a selfie with the main character, Owen. I unlocked my bike and rolled it past a few assistants, breaking down the lights and cables for the day. I stopped in front of the pizza shop to see my freshly showered Dad leaning against the menu board.

"Thanks for coming. I really appreciate it," Dad said.

"You've been trying to get a hold of me since the movie started. I figured you are probably heading back to Los Angeles now that the movie is almost done."

"You figured right. Are you hungry?"

Dad had two slices of pizza on a plate and handed me one slice. His first bite consumed half the slice. I handed my slice back to Dad while I pulled my insulin pump out of my pocket. Judging by the size of the large slice I figured it had about fifty carbohydrates in it. I had to guess the nutritional number since most of these boardwalk restaurants did not post their nutritional information. I punched the number of carbs into my device, and the insulin was instantly delivered. No needles, no waiting before eating. I slipped the small pump back into my pocket and took my first bite. Dad watched me intently the whole time.

"So, that is how the pump works? How are you doing with the diabetes?"

I continued chewing. "Well, Dad. I still have it, and I will continue to have it until a cure is found."

"I'm sorry I wasn't really around much for all of that."

"You weren't around at all. When things got tough, you took off to Hollywood!"

I was getting angry when I told myself to stay calm. I told myself I would be more positive when I thought the pier was going to explode with me on it.

Dad started raising his voice in response to mine. "I was chasing my dream. Don't you have dreams?"

"I do have dreams, Dad. Lots of them. But your whole family could have helped you with your dreams of acting. You didn't have to just walk away. You could have acted around here and not gone all the way to Hollywood. And now you are back here only because of the movie and not because of me."

"I want to see you more," Dad said. "You are older now, more mature. I want to be more involved in your future. I want to make up for so much lost time."

I didn't know how to respond. My brain was sizzling like overcooked bacon. Maybe I really did need to see my therapist more often and have her crazy cat, Mr. Cuddles, stare at me suspiciously. I was boiling on the inside, and I knew raising my stress level was not good for my diabetes. It was downright dangerous.

"Dad. I don't think you can make up for lost time. I'm just not sure about any future between us."

Dad didn't say anything. I didn't expect him to. He was always good at yelling and getting angry. He was never very good at politely verbalizing what was going on inside his head. I tossed the pizza crust into a trash barrel, unlocked my bike, and put on my helmet. I gave Dad a firm handshake.

"Goodbye, Dad. I have your number. We'll text when I'm ready."

I peddled away and left Dad holding his half-eaten pizza. I just shook off one zombie and felt a bit lighter now.

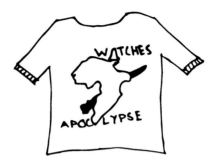

CHAPTER FIFTEEN
A Fresh Start

In many states, Labor Day weekend signals the start of a new school year and the official end of summer. I lamented over the things that I didn't get to do this summer. I never went to an amusement park, and I didn't get to eat enough ice cream. The list was pretty short, so maybe I was being selfish about my summer in a nutshell.

I paid Squirrel his share once the movie company sent me my last check. Mom and I went down to the bank and opened a savings account for me. She refused to take any of the money I earned to help her with our groceries, internet, or rent. Just last week, Mom and Dad spoke for almost an hour to flesh out a new plan. Dad was serious about trying to be a part of my present and future. His payout for the movie was quite substantial, and he agreed to send Mom a check once a month that would almost cover our rent. Mom did not want to get lawyers involved and was relieved to be getting something for the first time ever.

Mom took me out for dinner to celebrate receiving Dad's first check. I had not been to a posh restaurant with her in ages. It was one of those places with cloth napkins, unlimited bread baskets, and you didn't even have crayons at the table. I even had to wear dress pants to the dinner, no cargo shorts. I was a bit nervous, and Mom told me to only butter a small piece of the bread at one time and not smother the entire slice with butter. I tried not to be a Neanderthal the entire night. By the end, I was tired, but Mom even let me order dessert. After we came back from dinner, Mom covered my eyes and walked me by the hand into my bedroom. I slowly opened my eyes to see the new bedroom set she had delivered while we were out. It was a new bed and desk. My room received an enormous upgrade, and I was now ready for middle school.

Dad texted me a few times after he landed back in Los Angeles. Mom was afraid he was going to blow up my data usage. He even sent me his limited-edition zombie action figure, the same one I saw at Smiley's Comics. I hadn't opened the box, but it was sitting on my new desk. At least I didn't throw it out. He was taking more acting classes, and he received a small part in an upcoming superhero TV show. I texted him back with a "cool beans" response. It was short and sweet, and I did not elaborate on what I was doing or how I was feeling about sixth grade about to start. He didn't get that kind of insider access yet. I was going to take it real slow.

Exuberant bus driver Merle was pleased to see me when I was back on his morning route heading north out of Salem toward the Flowing Meadows School.

"Same stop, Mr. Zander?" Merle asked.

"Yes, Merle, drop me right at downtown and then just a short walk to school. Mr. Merle, I am starting middle school this morning."

"Excellent, Mr. Zander, you are moving up in the world. Probably more responsibility and a mountain of homework. Did you have a good summer?"

I told Merle a few of the events, but I did not detail all of them. I mentioned I had a part in the Salem zombie movie.

Merle let out a huge groan when I mentioned the movie.

"That movie? Traffic was a nightmare all summer because of that silly horror movie. I guess I will have to see it now that I drive a movie star to school every day."

I closed the journal that Dr. Storm had given me. During the last few days, I'd started to record some of my thoughts about my disease and how the last few years had gone. It felt good to get some of the buzzing out of my brain and down on paper. I felt my phone vibrate. It was a text from Squirrel. I opened it to see that Squirrel was sending me cartoon characters with their tongues sticking out because he still had two more days of summer left, and I was starting today. I clicked on his next message. Squirrel showed me an early design for a Witches Apocalypse t-shirt he designed. It was a cool logo for the movie with a picture of Zombie Dad choking me at the pier. I tried to forget the whole moment, but there it was right on a t-shirt. Somehow, in between stealing snacks from the film crew and bothering actors, Squirrel had snapped a fantastic shot of the ending scene on the pier. He then turned that photo into a graphically cool shirt.

Squirrel wrote in his third text, "We are going to sell these shirts downtown for twenty-five dollars a pop starting October first. We will make a killing from the Halloween tourists and with the movie coming out, it will be a hit. Money in the bank. Easy peasy. Are you in?"

I reread Squirrel's text one more time. He was already off on his next money-making scheme. Except this time, it seemed thought out and reasonable. Squirrel definitely had the money-making plan ready. Why not make some more money off the film and my dad?

"Sure," I texted back. "I am in."

He texted back immediately. He must have his device surgically attached to him while I was on this bus.

"Great. We make ten dollars each in profit on every shirt. I will even split the profit fifty-fifty on this project since it is your strangled neck on the shirt. Book all your weekends in October to start selling and put on your cheerful face for the tourists," texted Squirrel.

I always needed a friend like Squirrel to push me along even when I didn't want to be pushed. Working a t-shirt cart with him sounded like a new adventure.

Merle dropped me off at my bus stop in downtown North Beverly, and I walked my familiar route to school. I felt good wearing a new backpack, shiny sneakers, and dress shorts. I was able to keep my blood-soaked cargo shorts and hat, but those two items were tucked away in my closet waiting for next summer's movie premiere. Squirrel would probably put the clothing to good use and try to auction it as movie memorabilia for a high price next summer.

I walked into the Middle School building and checked out my new locker.

The opened locker slammed shut next to me.

"Hi Zander, long time," Cynthia said with a smile.

I took a big gulp.

"I heard about your big scene on the bridge. I can't wait to see the movie next summer."

"With me?" I asked.

"Of course, silly. We need a do-over after the museum situation. Hopefully we can get together again much sooner than the movie premiere."

"I hope so too." It was all I could squeak out.

"How have you been feeling?" she asked.

I lifted a piece of my shirt to show her my new pump.

"Cool new tech, Zander. I'm impressed," Cynthia responded.

"Oh yeah, about the museum. What happened there won't happen again. Trust me," I promised her.

Another locker slammed shut.

"Trust this guy? Are you kidding me?"

I turned around to see Brady heading toward us.

"Are you two hanging out now? Cynthia, you are joking right? Didn't I text you about all the awards I won this summer? I will tell you over lunch. Did Zander tell you about his participation award in our race together?"

"Not yet, Brady. I will see you at lunch, Zander."

Cynthia walked past me and totally dismissed Brady.

I showed a few classmates my insulin pump and how it worked.

Some were a tad grossed out by the tube attached to my stomach, but I just shrugged it off. After eating with Cynthia, I walked across the courtyard to see my new friend. I greeted the school receptionist as I headed down the hallway to the Lower School classrooms. The first few days of school were one of the few times a student could see a reflection on the floor. The cleanliness was almost palpable. I slowly peeked my head into the first-grade room to see students eating their lunches at their little desks and tiny chairs. I let my head loiter in the doorway until I made eye contact with him.

A classmate tapped Billy on the shoulder, and he whipped his body around. Billy gave me a big wave and smiled from ear to ear. He was eating his lunch at his table group. I was about to pull my head away from the doorway when Billy held up a finger signaling me to wait. He put his sandwich down and lifted the bottom of his shirt a little to reveal a tiny insulin pump and a tube coming out of it and attached to his stomach.

Billy cupped his hands together and while his teacher was still giving lunchtime instructions, he whispered loudly, "It's the same as yours!"

I lifted the bottom of my shirt to show my pump hooked onto the belt buckle of my shorts as well. We both gave each other the thumbs up, and I ducked out of the doorway. I headed back down the hallway, gave a head nod to Murse Liam, and walked out into the school's courtyard. The early September midday sun was blasting down on me, and it felt good. "Stay positive," I said to no one in particular.

I had to do quite a bit of checking up this school year. I was adding Billy to my "checking up" list. I had to check up on him, Mom, occasionally Dad, Squirrel, my therapist, and her cat. I had to keep checking in on my diabetes, and I would be ready for whatever came next.